WHAT EVERYONE SHOULD KNOW ABOUT DRUGS

Overcoming Common Problems

Other books in the same series

Overcoming Common Problems

WHAT EVERYONE SHOULD KNOW ABOUT DRUGS

Kenneth Leech

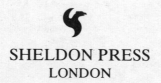

SHELDON PRESS

LONDON

First published in Great Britain in 1983 by
Sheldon Press, SPCK, Marylebone Road, London NW1 4DU

British Library Cataloguing in Publication Data

Leech, Kenneth
  What everyone should know about drugs.—
  (Overcoming common problems)
  1. Drugs—Physiological effect
  I. Title   II. Series
  615'.7   RM300

  ISBN 0-85969-382-1
  ISBN 0-85969-374-0 Pbk

Typeset by Memo Typography Ltd
Nicosia, Cyprus
Printed in Great Britain by
Richard Clay (The Chaucer Press) Ltd
Bungay, Suffolk.

Contents

'Nowhere in the world are there elders who know what their children know, no matter how remote and simple the societies are in which the children live... Once the fact of a deep new unprecedented world-wide generation gap is firmly established in the minds of both the young and the old, communications can be established again.'

MARGARET MEAD

Preface

I got involved in working with young drug addicts in 1964, more or less by accident, and have been involved, to varying degrees, with problems of young people and drugs ever since. To examine the complex issues which arise in this field would require a much more detailed book than this one. But there is a need for a simple book, addressed primarily to parents, which assumes little knowledge, and which seeks to present the essential facts about young people and drug abuse. That is what I have tried to do.

At various points I have quoted individual cases. In all of these, the names and details have been altered. So, while they are based on actual people, none of the individuals can be recognized from the descriptions.

K.L.   1983

1

Fact versus Fiction

All of us, whether we are parents, children, or whoever we are, are confronted constantly with a mass of 'information' about the dangers of drugs. The press bombards us with horror stories and warnings, and, even though there will be periods, sometimes several years, when other issues take over from drugs, the continuing story of 'the drugs menace' is always resumed. Yet on no other subject is there so much propaganda, so much hysteria. Indeed, it seems at times that when facts contradict fiction, it is the facts which are regarded as suspect. A whole industry of 'disinformation' has grown up around drugs and drug abuse, and if we are to reach any kind of sensible conclusions about the issues, we have to start cutting our way through the mass of myths, half-truths and untruths. In this book I have tried to approach the vast subject of drug abuse as calmly and reasonably as I can. It is hard to be calm and reasonable when one's closest friends, perhaps one's own children, are involved. We feel helpless and confused, not only by the situation, but also by the bewildering range of conflicting views and opinions. Complete objectivity is not possible, and there will continue to be differing views on many of the questions, for it is a vast field, a complex field, and, in many respects, a new field. Let us start by looking at some of the widespread, yet false, assumptions which are made about drugs.

'Drugs mainly affect young people'

Even well-informed people often assume that most drug problems involve the young, that most drug misusers, abusers and addicts (for definition of these terms see p. 43) are young, and that it is the young who consume most harmful drugs. Yet this is completely mistaken. Most drug problems involve middle-aged

1

and elderly people. Most drug misusers, abusers and addicts come in the middle-aged and elderly groups. It is the middle-aged and elderly who consume most harmful drugs, indeed most drugs of any kind. Young people may use different drugs, though this is not always the case. The fact is that we are a drug-using society. For years we have accepted the principle of 'better living through chemistry'; the principle that the best way to solve our *internal* problems is to do something *externally*. Whatever is wrong with us — headache, depression, anxiety, loneliness, lack of meaning — there must be a pill somewhere which will solve the problem. This is not something which young people have invented; in fact, many young people have rebelled against our excessive reliance on chemical solutions. It is adults who consume the vast amounts of alcohol, tranquillizers, anti-depressants, sedatives, and so on, which are pushed at us by firms, doctors and the media. So there is nothing very surprising if young people, brought up in this drug-saturated society, take drugs to solve their problems: it is the most natural thing to do, it is what they have been taught by adults to do. It would be very odd if there were no drug problems among the young!

Of course, the drugs which adults take have less news value than those taken by young people. But that does not mean that they are less dangerous or less addictive. One of the greatest problems in the West is the growing number of people who have become dependent on sedative and tranquillizer drugs. These drugs have for the most part been produced since the last war, but in the last fifteen years their use has increased dramatically. Many millions of prescriptions are issued for such drugs as Librium, Mogadon and Valium. Between 1966 and 1977 there was a 75 per cent increase in prescriptions for anti-depressants and tranquillizers, and a 200 per cent increase in prescriptions for hypnotic (that is, sleep-inducing) drugs, other than the barbiturates. There has been a good deal of research into the use of drugs to curb anxiety, and it is clear that the majority of users are women aged 25—34 and 45—54.

Again, if we take the commonest drug of all, alcohol, it is clear

2

TABLE 1

Diagram Showing Percentage Change In Prescriptions Of Mind-Altering Drugs In UK 1966-77

Percentage Change

+200
+150
+100
+50
0
-50

66 67 68 69 70 71 72 73 74 75 76 77

non-barbiturate hypnotics

antidepressants
tranquillizers

stimulants
barbiturate hypnotics

that it is not the young who form the bulk of abusers or alcoholics. So in confronting the 'drug problem', we are confronting a problem which afflicts many sections of our society, but particularly the middle-aged and elderly.

'Drugs are mainly illegal, illegally produced and illegally distributed'

Again, this is simply incorrect. Most drugs which are used are perfectly legal, manufactured by reputable companies, prescribed by doctors, dispensed by chemists. While there are illegal drugs, the biggest drug-abuse problem is a legal problem. Let us take alcohol again as an example. This book will for the most part deal with drugs other than alcohol, but we need to remember that alcohol is a drug of addiction, and that it leads to more serious problems than all the illegal drugs put together. Alcohol is perfectly legal (as indeed are tobacco and benzodiazepines). A visitor from Mars would be surprised to find that a drug which was so dangerous that around two per cent of the earth's population was permanently incapacitated by its use was freely available in licensed distribution centres (pubs), while other equally or less dangerous substances were outlawed. We are not very consistent. Of course, most alcoholics are not young people, but there is a growing body of evidence that more young people are turning to alcohol as a drug of abuse. A study in Scotland has suggested that as many as forty per cent of adolescents may be on the road to alcoholism. In a study of patients in a general practice of 3,000, it has been claimed that there will be around thirty heavy drinkers, twenty-seven for whom drink has become a problem, and twenty-seven who are addicted to alcohol.

Most of the drugs other than alcohol which are abused, whether by young people or older people, are also legal, though there may be legal controls on their distribution and use. Barbiturates, amphetamines, sedatives, tranquillizers, even heroin and cocaine, are manufactured and prescribed within the law. Compared with the vast numbers of legally available drugs, those which are of illegal origin are only a small proportion of the total.

'Drugs are controlled by criminal syndicates and pushers'

There is some truth in this view which has been widely promoted by the sensationalist press for years. In recent years the criminal syndicates have moved in increasingly on certain areas of the drug scene. But again it is essential not to be misled by horror stories of gangsters and pushers. Most drugs do not come from pushers but from doctors and chemists who have prescribed and dispensed them with quite legitimate intent. Even those who use illegal drugs often obtain them from friends and acquaintances. Addiction spreads more through person-to-person contact than through any sinister conspiracy. The picture of the pusher, lurking in darkened alleyways, ready to ensnare the innocent child and make him or her an addict against his or her will, owes more to fantasy than to reality.

Even where illegal drugs are involved, or where a legally obtained drug is then distributed illegally, most people only come into contact with their *immediate* source of supply (i.e. the small-scale pusher). Nor is the picture of the entirely innocent, passive child, who is made into an addict against his will, a correct one. Apart from the small numbers of people who become addicted by accident as a result of having a drug prescribed for treatment ('therapeutic addicts'), almost all drug addicts or drug abusers have made a conscious choice to use the drug. None of this is to deny the existence of Mafias and similar organized criminal groupings: but to focus on them can easily shift attention away from the much more serious problems of respectable, legal drug abuse, and, in any case, the ordinary addict in the street does not come across them for the most part.

'Drugs are all equally dangerous'

Again, this is simply untrue, and to tell such a serious untruth to young people can easily undermine their credibility in all drug information which emanates from adults. It is just as ridiculous to say that drugs are harmless. No drug is free from harm. Most drugs can be abused, and even the most commonly used drugs, such as aspirin or paracetamol, can kill. A lot depends on the dosage, the circumstances in which the drug is taken, the condition of the person who takes it, and so on. Yet there are levels of danger and of harm, and some drugs are less dangerous than others. For example, it is inaccurate and irresponsible to place cannabis in the same category as heroin. If adults continue to tell intelligent young people of the terrible dangers of cannabis smoking in such a way that no distinction is made between one drug and another, they will soon lose confidence in all adult 'facts' about drugs. It is a classic 'cry wolf' situation. Fortunately today there is a decline in the readiness of many people to identify the two drugs in this simplistic way.

Very often the most dangerous drugs are those which attract least attention in the press and in our own thinking. Take the barbiturates, which were until recently the most widely used sleeping pills. More people were dying throughout the 1960s every week in England and Wales alone from barbiturates than have been shown to have died from cannabis in the entire history of the human race! Yet the press told us more about the horrors of 'pot' than about these respectable sleeping tablets. Alcohol is a killer drug, far more lethal than heroin and far more destructive. For a number of years I worked in a centre in Soho which ran a referral clinic for heroin users in part of the building which was also regularly visited by vagrant alcoholics. Many times a week one saw how much more destructive were the physical and social effects of alcohol than were those of heroin. Yet one drug was respectable and the other was taboo. (Of course, the *percentage* of alcohol users who are seriously damaged is much less than that of heroin users, but the *numbers* are much higher.)

Again, we know that even the really dangerous and addictive drugs in most cases have their own uses and limited value. Heroin is used to good effect in treating terminal cancer pain. Other powerful pain killers have their value in treatment but can become drugs of addiction. Many people are only alive today because of the right use of potentially dangerous drugs. So we need to be careful not to dismiss all drugs as dangerous and to ignore the great value and benefits which drugs have brought, and still bring, to mankind.

Finally, many of the dangers which people associate with drugs are actually dangers which belong to the life-style of drug takers more than to the drug itself. There is the world of difference between the clean and careful administration of a drug in a hospital setting, and street drug use which may involve dirty needles, lack of food and accommodation, malnutrition, abscesses, and so on. The majority of deaths of heroin addicts have as much to do with the life-style and the factors linked with drug use as with the drug itself. In fact, it is often the weakest drug (in terms of addictive potential) which is the most dangerous. Street heroin sold in New York City usually contains so little heroin that in order to become addicted to the heroin one must consume massive amounts of powder. But it is the very impurity and adulteration of the powdered drug which makes it so dangerous to life. While thousands of deaths in the city are attributed to heroin overdose, research has shown that this is not usually the cause of death at all.

'Most people start on soft drugs and then go on to hard drugs'

This is a widely held view, but a misleading one. For a start, the distinction between 'soft' and 'hard' drugs is not a very helpful one. Sometimes people mean by this distinction that some drugs are physically addictive and others are not. But often drugs which can cause physical addiction are put in the 'soft' category, while less dangerous ones are termed 'hard'. In any case, physical addiction is not the only danger there is in drug use. It is better to drop the simple division between 'soft' and 'hard'. A more realistic distinction is that between those who inject and those who do not. But the patterns of drug use are so complex, and the ways in which drugs are used in a particular culture so different, that it is impossible to make simple distinctions which hold good for every situation.

When people think about 'progression' or 'escalation', what they have in mind is that young people start on a relatively harmless drug (such as cannabis) but soon progress to a more dangerous drug (such as heroin). There is some truth in this stepping-stone view, but it is also dangerously misleading. The truth is that most (but not all) heroin addicts have in the past used cannabis and various pills. It is probably also true that most methylated spirit drinkers have at some point drunk beer. But this is to say no more than that, if you are part of a drug-using culture, you are more likely to move to more dangerous drugs or more dangerous use of the same drugs than if you are not part of such a culture at all. The point is that most beer drinkers do *not* become methylated spirit addicts or alcoholics of any kind. Similarly most cannabis users or pilltakers do *not* become heroin addicts or addicts of any kind. If they did, we would have millions of drug addicts in Britain today.

As in other areas, a good deal depends on the district, the culture, the availability of drugs, the individual, and so on. Thus on a world scale, one finds areas like the Caribbean where cannabis and alcohol are widely used but where more dangerous opiate drugs are unknown, and other areas such as Hong Kong where heroin use is endemic but cannabis is not widely used. Within Britain, patterns of drug use vary greatly. Take the following four examples of young people who have used cannabis.

Derek: a young working-class drug addict. Began to use amphetamines in early teens and smoked cannabis. Later used heroin and became addicted. Still uses a variety of injectible drugs. No longer smokes cannabis much, but injects whatever injectible drugs he can buy on the black market.

Tony: went to public school. Cannabis was in circulation so he began to smoke. No other drugs were available or in vogue other than alcohol. Very conventional young man, and when cannabis went out of fashion in his circle, he stopped. Knows nothing of addiction, has never met a heroin user, and does not consider himself a part of any drug scene.

Steve: was part of a 'hippy' culture where cannabis and LSD were an integral part of the life-style. But the hippy culture was strongly opposed to needle drugs and expressed its disapproval. Steve used LSD a few times, found it helpful, but has not used it now for years. He still smokes cannabis recreationally with friends. No other drug use.

Delroy: young man of West Indian parentage. Rastafarian. Smokes cannabis regularly and considers it an important part of the Rasta culture. Also drinks in moderation. Has never used any other drugs, has no interest in, or knowledge of, needle drugs.

These four young people have less in common with each other than the fact that they all have used cannabis might lead the innocent outside observer to believe. They come from totally different backgrounds, and within these backgrounds they began to use cannabis. For Derek, cannabis, along with amphetamines, violence, taking and driving away of vehicles, and truancy, was part of the accepted environment in which he grew up. It was as natural that he would use that drug as that he would steal from the local store. He quickly moved to more powerful drugs which seemed to answer his very deep emotional needs. For Tony, cannabis was simply part of the trend in his school at a particular time. Being an extremely conventional young man, he followed the trend while it lasted. He is now just as conventional, and has moved over to the recreational use of alcohol. Steve belonged to a group of gentle, non-violent people who rarely came into conflict with the law and would not have done so at all had it not been for the illegal status of the drugs of their choice. But, like his friends, he was always opposed to the use of amphetamines and heroin. It was simply not the done thing in that culture, any more than it was in Delroy's.

There is therefore no automatic progression from one drug to another. Some progress, some stay with one drug, some give up altogether. In some areas, a wide range of drugs circulates within the same streets. Elsewhere this is not the case. Whether people move from one drug to another depends on many different factors. But we should realize that there is a lot of evidence to show that, while some people 'escalate', others 'de-escalate', that is, they use less and less amounts of drugs, and may give up altogether. Much drug use is a passing trend, and it may give way to other, perhaps more harmful, trends. At one time I worked in a part of London with a very high delinquency rate. On certain estates one could almost guarantee that the younger members of some families would be using drugs of the amphetamine type. Ten years later, I went back to the same estates. No longer were amphetamines, or any other drugs (other than alcohol), part of the fashion. The young teenagers instead were joining the National Front campaign and were involved in attacks on Asians. Some progress!

'Once an addict, always an addict'

The truth behind this view is the undoubted fact that addiction to drugs such as heroin, and involvement in a 'needle culture', is an extremely difficult life-style to break with. It gets a grip on people which is so powerful that they find it very hard to split from both the drug and the culture. However, not all drug takers are addicted, not all drugs have the same effects, and many of those who have become addicted to dangerous drugs do in fact come off. Take the following cases of young people, all of whom were at one time heavily involved in the drug culture of the West End of London.

Sheila: was once on heroin, intravenous amphetamine, and a variety of other drugs. Has now been off for over fifteen years. Occasional relapses, usually associated with some crisis in her personal life.

Cathy: was on heroin for three years and at the centre of a particular group of musicians who all used drugs. Suddenly the prospect for the future terrified her, and she came off immediately without treatment. Has now been married, and off all drugs, for over ten years.

Ann: was very heavily addicted to heroin and barbiturates. Many 'cures' and periods in hospital, several long stretches in prison. Finally came off in hospital, and spent several years in a residential community. Now a teacher, and has been off all drugs for years.

Peter: was a 'pillhead' (high dose amphetamine user) and the key figure in a Soho club where amphetamines circulated. After several years he simply stopped, without treatment, and is now living a settled life in the suburbs.

These are not exceptional cases. Research both in the United States and Britain has shown that many addicts simply stop using drugs around the age of 30–35. The Americans call it 'maturing out'. Of course, there are others for whom life is short. After a few years on drugs, they overdose and die. And there are those who remain addicted for life. But not all do. One of the difficulties in this area is that many of those who simply stop using drugs do not keep in contact with their former associates or with therapeutic agencies: they simply disappear from view, and start a new life. It is probably best that they do break off all contacts from their past. There are probably thousands of such people, an invisible ex-addict population. They have no news value, and we tend to forget they are there.

'Drug addicts are violent criminals'

There is evidence to connect certain drugs with violence. This is particularly true in the case of alcohol and the barbiturates. But not all who use these drugs become violent; some become drowsy, silly and quiescent. What is probably true is that the drugs bring out the latent violence which is already present in some

11

people. Amphetamine, which is a very powerful stimulant, is often linked with violence. But there is little evidence to connect cannabis with violence, in spite of the derivation of 'assassin' from hashish. Many cannabis users are rather quiet, dreamy people, and heavy use is more likely to lead to cumulative lethargy than to violence.

Heroin does not produce violence either, nor do heroin addicts commit violent crimes under its influence. However, when heroin addicts are deprived of heroin, they may commit crimes in order to get money to buy further supplies of the drug. It is not heroin which produces crime, but the need for heroin which forces people to commit crime. But this can be overstated. Thus it is often said that heroin addicts are responsible for most of the crimes of property in New York City. Figures vary from 25 to 90 per cent. However, a study in 1974 by the Crime Analysis Unit of New York City Police Department showed that property crimes of arrested criminal heroin users and non-users were about the same, but that the percentage of non-users who committed serious crimes against the person was much higher than that of heroin users. A study by the Hudson Institute showed even lower figures: less than two per cent of addicts supported their heroin use by robbery or mugging. But, whatever the figures, undoubtedly some heroin addicts commit property crimes, not as a result of taking heroin, but as a result of the high cost of obtaining it on the American black market. In Britain, studies by members of the Home Office Research Unit have shown that heroin is more likely to lead to passive behaviour than to violent crime.

While the relation between drugs and crime is not simple, it is clear that the laws on drugs can produce criminals. Studies in prison have shown that where first offenders who have been sent to prison for possession of cannabis are, through imprisonment, brought into contact with the criminal world, the risk of further involvement may be increased. But this is not a matter of drugs leading to crime, but of prison leading to crime! Bad laws, or laws which are administered badly, may cause greater damage and more problems than the drugs against which they are aimed.

There are many false ideas which are widely held about drugs. Many of them are fostered by sections of the media who are more concerned with sensational stories than with the truth. So, if we are to separate drug fact from fiction, here is a maxim with which to begin:

Suspect the media

From the 1960s onwards sections of the British press have done incalculable harm by their treatment of drug issues. Seemingly unconcerned with facts or the results of research, they have been concerned more to propagate scare stories, to sensationalize, and to reinforce popular prejudices, punitive attitudes and ill-founded ideas. Often they have done this, as they do with their sordid treatment of sexuality, with a spurious high moral tone, claiming that they are the guardians of the nation's purity, and similar nonsense. This is not to deny that, in the same period, a small minority of well-informed and socially responsible journalists have done a great deal to help create an educated public on drug issues. But, as a whole, it is wise not to trust the popular media as a reliable guide to facts about drugs. Approach them always with a high level of suspicion and caution.

Studies of the ways in which myths and prejudices are propagated by press coverage contain horrifying examples. Thus, while everyone who has worked in the field of drug abuse, and anyone who has read any piece of serious research on the subject, knows that it is simply not true that most cannabis users 'escalate' to heroin, this view has been churned out over and over again in the mass media. But many of the myths are less crude than this. Often a newspaper will make drugs to be the central feature of a story in order to increase its news value even though a careful study shows that the drug element was negligible or disputed. Thus one paper had headlines 'Drug crazed man raped young nurse twice'. Study of the case showed that the judge had given no credence to the claim that the rapist was 'crazed' on LSD, a claim which had been used by the young man as a defence for his action. 'Thirty registered LSD addicts in Northampton' announced a local paper in 1972, although LSD is not addictive, and there is not, and never has been, any system of registration of its users.

LSD has produced some of the worst examples of press handling of drug cases. Reports of genetic damage have been reproduced as if they were the confirmed results of research. The LSD-taker who, believing he could fly, jumped from a high-rise flat, has become part of drug mythology even though nobody has ever produced any evidence for his existence. Thus one paper in 1978 announced:

> Takers have been known to leap off buildings believing they could fly...chew a hand down to the bone believing it to be an orange...or truss and prepare a baby for roasting, believing it to be an oven-ready chicken.

By contrast, the well-documented studies of LSD use present a very different kind of picture.

It is never wise to rely on the press for information on the details of drug use. While there are many careful and thorough reporters who check their facts scrupulously, this is not always the case. A recent example was the question of deaths as a result of glue-sniffing. On 3 April 1981, a question was asked in the House of Commons on the number of deaths from glue-sniffing. Sir George Young replied that exact figures on *solvent* abuse were not available. (Solvents include compounds contained not only in glue but in paints, nail varnish remover, dry cleaning fluids, degreasing compounds, etc.) Earlier, on 12 March, he had given a figure of 22 known deaths in Great Britain in 1980, but on 3 April he apologized for the fact that this was incorrect, and said that the correct figure was 13. However, on 13 October three papers repeated the earlier figure of 22 with headlines such as '22 deaths in glue-sniffing epidemic' and '22 die as glue-sniffing craze spreads'. Not only were the numbers wrong, but the deaths were from *solvent* abuse, not glue-sniffing alone. Most did not involve glue at all.

Another, more serious, example of misleading reporting on glue-sniffing occurred in February 1980 after an inquest on a boy of 17 who had died after sniffing glue. On 15 February one paper's headline was 'Boy, 17, died in cell after sniffing glue', while another on the 16th announced 'Boy "high on glue" died in police cell'. However, the inquest report shows that the boy had been arrested with five friends, all smelling of glue, and half a tube had been found on one of them. But the dead boy had also been using barbiturates for some time, and had taken twenty Tuinal tablets. The death certificate clearly states that the cause of death was barbiturate poisoning, not glue-sniffing.

The most worrying aspect of the role of the media is the way in which newspaper accounts can actually lead to an increase in certain kinds of drug abuse. We shall look in Chapter 4 at one example of this, also in connection with glue-sniffing. But there are many others. While the Press may be attacking certain drugs in such a way as to increase the likelihood of their use as well as reinforce inaccurate views about them, the same papers may at the same time be advertising other drugs, particularly alcohol, with no moral qualms at all.

If we need to suspect the media, a second maxim will be:

Be wary of crusaders

Crusaders are attracted to the drug scene as moths to a flame. Many of them are desperately sincere, dedicated men and women, who feel that God has called them to work in this area. Many others do not work in the field itself but speak about it. But the drug scene also attracts a number of unbalanced, fanatical people, who find that they can use such work as a way of working through their own personal problems. Many of these people have an extrovert, flamboyant, sensation-loving temperament, not unlike the mass media. They will speak and write in highly emotional language, perhaps make films and write books which describe their work in very dramatic ways. Unfortunately they rarely have much sense of factual accuracy, and it is possible to be led astray by their sincerity and zeal into believing that what they are saying is factually true. They are prone to gross exaggeration, and often pay no attention to the results of research. So be wary of crusaders, and recognize that, while they may have close links with drug users, they are often among the most unreliable commentators on what is happening. Of course, as patterns of drug use develop, more responsible people tend to replace these crusaders who are more evident in the early days of the drug scene. However, many people of the moral crusading type continue to use 'the drug menace' as part of their campaigning material, though their contact with drug users may be slight or non-existent.

Beware of drug manufacturers' claims

Drugs are manufactured by multi-national companies with vast resources and elaborate advertising techniques. While there is no doubt that modern drugs have been of great value in making life tolerable and in curing disease, it is also the case that some drug companies have exploited personal and social problems, and have often been dishonest about their claims and about the effects of their products. Many adverts are both inaccurate and unethical. They make claims for the unique and precise effect of a drug which independent research does not support. They often ignore harmful side-effects. Some suggest an instant cure when this is clearly not the case. Doctors are bombarded with propaganda from drug companies extolling the virtues of their products. Some of the worst tragedies of the 1960s were the result of the production of centrally acting drugs by certain companies, although independent research had shown these products to be more dangerous than useful.

In general, it can be said that the effectiveness of a drug is in inverse proportion to the amount spent on advertising it. The amount spent on advertising drugs is probably greater than that spent on research. Of course, many doctors exercise a degree of caution and suspicion in relation to drug companies' claims. But

16

the pressures are considerable. Some notable medical figures are paid advisers to drug companies, while some medical journals depend on drug companies' adverts for their survival. So beware of some of the claims made by drug companies. They are often wide of the mark, and motivated by profit rather than truth.

This chapter has been to a large extent depressing. I have warned of the danger of taking people at their face value, and of the exaggerated and inaccurate claims made by drug manufacturers. The point is that drugs are big business, but it is respectable business for the most part. As parents and people concerned with rescuing young people from harm, we are up against greater odds than are apparent at first sight. For this is a drug culture, a society dominated by drugs and claims made for drugs. We need to cut through the mass of disinformation, and reach the truth which is so often buried beneath the mountains of prejudice, untruth and propaganda. In doing this we need to beware of making our own sweeping judgements, to be suspicious of ourselves.

Finally, we need to try to keep up to date. The drug scene is always changing and so is drug research. It is easy to get out of date and out of touch. However, the motivations of drug users are probably not all that different from one generation to another, and it is wrong for parents and teachers to assume that drug abuse among the young is so novel and idiosyncratic that it is outside their experience entirely. Parents can understand a lot of what they need to know about their children's drug habits by making connections with their own experiences, for example, with alcohol, cigarettes or prescribed medicines. At the same time, we should accept the limitations of our knowledge and be willing to learn from young people what they can teach us.

2

Young People and Drugs

The word 'drug' originated by mistake. It grew from the Low German *drog vate*, meaning 'dry casks', and it was used, wrongly, to describe the contents, although the word 'drog' simply meant 'dry'. From this curious origin, the word came to be used of the contents of the casks. In this book we are concerned with what are in fact a small range of drugs, those which affect the central nervous system (CNS), i.e. the brain, and particularly the minority of these drugs which are abused by young people. Not all drugs affect the CNS and not all those which do become 'drugs of abuse'. It is important to remember this, and to resist the temptation to attack all drugs indiscriminately.

What is a drug? The World Health Organization (WHO) has defined it as 'any substance that, when taken into the living organism, may modify one or more of its functions'. Some drugs are contained in naturally occurring plants, and these have been used a good deal in folk medicine, as well as for recreational and religious purposes. But in recent years a whole new world of synthetic drugs has grown up, and the sciences of pharmacology (the study of drug action) and pharmacy (the preparation of drugs for use in medicine) have become essential parts of modern science. However, there is much that we do not know about the precise nature of drug action. The human brain is itself a complex chemical system. So when we introduce drugs into ourselves, we are introducing one chemical into a system of chemicals. By doing this, we establish a two-way relationship. Drugs affect personality, but the personality of the user also affects the drug. Different people are affected by a drug in different ways.

Of course, there are many drugs which do not affect the central nervous system at all because they cannot enter it from the bloodstream. There is a blood—brain barrier which allows only certain types of molecules to enter the brain. However, a fever may alter

TABLE 2

Table of main drugs discussed

1	Stimulants	Main types	Nicknames
		Amphetamines and	
		Amphetamine compounds	
		e.g. Dexedrine	dex, dexies
		Drinamyl	blues, purple hearts (old name)
		Durophet	black bombers
		Methedrine	meth
		Others: Preludin	
		Cocaine	coke
		Tenuate Ritalin	
2	Cannabis	Hashish (resin)	hash
		Marijuana or ganja (from flowering leaves and stem)	weed, grass, pot
		Cannabis oil	
		Synthetic THC	
3	LSD and psychedelics	LSD-25	acid
		PCP, DMT, etc.	
		Morning Glory seeds	
		Psilocybin and hallucinogenic mushrooms	
4	Hypnotics, sedatives and tranquillizers	Barbiturates	
		e.g. Tuinal Seconal	
		Nembutal Amytal	
		Non-barbiturate hypnotics	
		e.g. Mandrax (no longer manufactured in UK)	
		Mogadon	
		Minor tranquillizers	
		(Benzodiazepines)	
		e.g. Valium Librium Ativan	
5	Heroin and opiates	Heroin	H, horse, smack
		Synthetic opiates	
		Dipipanone (Diconal)	
		Methadone (Physeptone)	
		Codeine Opiate powders	
6	Glues and solvents	glues, paints, dry-cleaning fluids, aerosols, fuels	

this barrier for a time and enable responses to be made to substances in the bloodstream. The effect of a drug is related to the place, or site, of its action. For example, the drug LSD seems to block the action of a substance in the brain called serotonin, and throws its system temporarily out of order. The drug chlorpromazine, commonly known under its trade name of Largactil, blocks the action of nor-adrenalin, (another brain chemical).

The drugs with which we shall be concerned in this book fall into six main categories:

1   Stimulants, such as amphetamine, which *increase* activity;

2   Cannabis, a relatively mild intoxicant;

3   Psychedelic drugs, such as LSD, which change perception of reality;

4   Hypnotics, sedatives and tranquillizers, which *reduce* activity and induce sleep;

5   Heroin and other opiates, drugs derived from opium;

6   Solvents and other substances contained in glues, aerosols, etc.

Although many people think that 'the drug problem' is new, this is not so. The use and abuse of drugs is ancient. Many ancient cultures used drugs for religious purposes, to aid meditation, or for ritual reasons. Opium is mentioned in Assyrian medical tablets from the seventh century BC as well as in the writings of Homer, Ovid, Virgil and Pliny the Elder. We find many references to drugs throughout history. In the last century, nitrous oxide ('laughing gas') was used by many people, including Coleridge, Southey and Josiah Wedgwood. Cannabis was widely used by doctors, including the physician-in-ordinary to Queen Victoria, Dr Russell Reynolds, as a cure for all kinds of ailments. Ether became endemic in Northern Ireland in the aftermath of a temperance crusade! However, the twentieth century, and particularly the period since the last war, has seen a drugs revolution.

Nearly ninety per cent of the drugs which are now being prescribed were not invented ten or fifteen years ago. So while there is no way of knowing whether drug abuse has actually increased in the last hundred years, or whether people have simply substituted one drug for another, it is clear that there is now a much wider range of manufactured drugs from which people can choose.

Let us look then at the main types of drug used by young people since the drug epidemics of the early 1960s to the present day.

1 Stimulants

Speed

'Speed Kills', a slogan which one still finds on walls in parts of some cities, did not refer to dangerous driving, but to the abuse of drugs of the amphetamine type. Amphetamines are stimulant drugs, and we know them under such trade names as Dexedrine and Methedrine. It was the manufacture of a pill called Drinamyl, a mixture of amphetamine and barbiturate, in 1951 which ushered in the 'pep pill' era, though it was some years before the drug became widely abused by teenagers. Drinamyl soon became known as 'purple heart' although it was actually blue and triangular, and in 1964, when its shape was changed, it became known generally as 'blues' or 'French blues'. (Not, as some youngsters thought, because there was anything French about it, but because the manufacturers were Smith, Kline and French Ltd.) Before teenagers discovered this drug in the early 60s, it was widely used to combat fatigue and as a slimming pill. In fact, the earliest crop of addicts consisted not of young people but of overweight, middle-aged women.

Although Drinamyl became the best known of the pep pills, amphetamine had been prepared towards the end of the nineteenth century. The Benzedrine inhaler was introduced in 1932, while methylamphetamine (Methedrine) had been used in psychiatry, in spinal anaesthesia, and as the best cure for post-

21

operative hiccups! One of the major uses of the amphetamine drugs was to increase wakefulness, and they were therefore valued by nurses, long-distance drivers, night workers (including prostitutes), and the armed forces, as well as those who suffered from the relatively rare condition called narcolepsy (a state of regular sleepiness for which amphetamine is still the best drug). But by the late 1930s it was realized that excessive use of the drug could bring about a psychotic condition similar to paranoid schizophrenia, and there were disturbing reports from Japan and Sweden in particular in the 1950s.

The amphetamine psychosis, as it is known, is a condition marked by paranoid delusions and often by vivid and frightening hallucinations, combined with confusion and general excitement. The condition is particularly marked when the drug is injected intravenously. High-dose amphetamine users ('pill-heads' or 'speed freaks') take the drug in massive doses to obtain maximum effect, 'the flash', and will remain awake and highly active for days. This period of agitation and excitement will be followed by the 'crash' or 'come down' with exhaustion, severe depression, and sleep followed by hunger and further depression. The cycle will then start again. It was the spread of high-dose amphetamine use which transformed the Haight—Ashbury district of San Francisco from a gentle, hippy community into a violent and dangerous area. In 1968 kids in Haight—Ashbury were injecting 1,000—5,000 milligrammes of amphetamine per day although the pharmacology textbooks said that 250 milligrammes was a lethal dose. It was about the same time that the 'speed scene' hit London.

One of the interesting and encouraging things that came out of the epidemic of injecting amphetamime was the way in which sections of the drug-taking community alerted their friends to the dangers. The 'Speed Kills' slogan was very successful in deterring many young people from using Methedrine. A notice issued by the advice agency Release in 1968, and widely circulated among young people remains one of the most succinct warnings against the drug (although it overstated some of the dangers).

SPEED KILLS

It is not widely known that the side effects of taking certain drugs can do as much damage as the drugs themselves. Amphetamines are not as safe as has been supposed, and there is growing concern on the scene about the widespread use of Methedrine.

The amphetamine Methedrine is a powerful drug which distorts the mental state. Although it is used clinically to cure such disorders as Parkinsonism, Epilepsy, Enuresis and Obesity, abuse of the drug can have lasting and devastating effects.

Methedrine is one of the most dangerous drugs around at the moment, and although it is less physically addictive than heroin, its prolonged use can cause very unpleasant conditions.

The most striking feature of someone who is habituated to methedrine is a paranoid psychosis with delusions and hallucinations which may be indistinguishable from paranoid schizophrenia. A Methedrine user feels persecuted — friends become enemies — voices of a persecutory nature may be heard, and the persecutors (real to the sufferer but totally imaginary) may be seen and attacked.

Methedrine taken for a prolonged length of time will stop a girl's periods and diminish sexual potency. There is a possibility of brain damage even after the use of the drug is discontinued, and the conditions mentioned earlier can happen sooner or later to anyone who shoots methedrine. In fact fixing any drug with unsterile needles can cause

> Septicaemia (blood poisoning)
> Tetanus (lockjaw)
> Jaundice
> Gangrene
> Abscesses
> Syphilis
> Gonorrhoea

For further information ring Release

SPEED KILLS

There is evidence that the propaganda campaign by this street agency was successful though its claims about brain damage and death are questionable.

Of course, most of the young people who got on to the 'pill scene' were mere experimenters, and it was a minority who got into high dose usage. It was a minority too who injected the drug, the majority taking the pills by mouth. However, since the early 1970s when doctors began to reduce their prescribing of amphetamines, more illegal amphetamine in powder form has been manufactured, and there has been an increase in the circulation and use (by injection) of this material. Of the legally manufactured pills, Drinamyl, Dexedrine, Methedrine (restricted since 1968) and Durophet have remained the favourites, though others become popular from time to time. As a result of greater awareness in the medical profession that these drugs are more dangerous than useful, there are now far fewer legal amphetamines in circulation, and doctors tend to prescribe safer drugs as alternatives. They are also now subject to stricter legal control.

However, it is unwise to assume that the amphetamine era is over. During the punk explosion of the late 1970s the drug was revived, and its use is a feature of 'disco' life and of the North of England's Soul club scene. Both legally produced pills and illicit powder are used. Again, while in the late 60s the principal concern was with the injection of amphetamine, there has in recent years been a revival of sniffing both amphetamine sulphate powder and cocaine.

Cocaine

The revival of cocaine use is particularly marked in, though by no means restricted to, the upper middle classes and fashionable groups on the London scene. Unlike its use in the 60s, when it was a companion drug to heroin and was injected, today cocaine is usually used by itself and by people who are not part of a needle culture. Amphetamines have tended to be associated with working-class young people, though again this is not to deny their use by other groups. With the reappearance of drug abuse among young people in a variety of areas, we have also seen a search for new, more easily obtainable, stimulants. One example is the popularity in some areas of the appetite-reducing agent Tenuate or Tenuate Dospan, prescribed widely for overweight. In fact, much illicit 'amphetamine' is actually diethylpropion hydrochloride (the active ingredient of Tenuate Dospan), not amphetamine at all.

2   Cannabis

Cannabis is not strictly a drug at all but a plant which sometimes produces drug effects. *Cannabis sativa* is the name of the hemp plant which grows throughout the world. From the flowering tops of the plant comes the drug know as marijuana (grass) or, in West Indian communities, ganja. From the resin comes hashish which is more potent, though in smoked form there is probably little difference. There are many slang terms for the cannabis drugs which vary from one cultural group to another, from place to place, and from time to time. In Britain, it is hashish ('hash') which is more common, though 'home grown' cannabis is increasingly popular and West Indians and Rastafarians much prefer grass. The drug has been used in eastern countries for many centuries — including its use in religious practice — and in cultures where alcohol is forbidden. In Britain it was widely used medicinally until this century. Culpepper's Herbal (1652) claimed that it was 'so well-known to every good housewife in the country that I shall not need to write any description of it'.

The smoking of cannabis in Britain began in ports and among merchant seamen from countries where the drug was common. It was also used by jazz musicians, poets and early beatnik and bohemian groups. Its spread to much wider sections of society occurred in the middle and late 60s, and today it would be impossible to speak of a 'typical' cannabis user. The drug is used by a very wide variety of people of differing age, social class, education and outlook. Many, probably most, of those who use cannabis have little if any contact with other drugs or with the 'drug culture'. However, simply because the only sources for the drug are illegal ones, there is a possibility that users will be brought into contact with criminal groups who may be able to supply them with more dangerous substances. Whether this occurs or not varies from place to place. The context in which the drug is used is so varied that it is not possible to generalize. However, whatever *might* happen, it is possible to say what, as a matter of fact, does not happen: most cannabis users do not enter the numbers of the heroin or narcotic addicts. (Cannabis is — misleadingly — still defined as a narcotic by the United Nations.) That much is clear from the statistics.

Cannabis is not itself an addictive drug and should not be linked with drugs like heroin with which it has nothing in common. In the form in which it circulates, it is not at all a powerful drug, and the best description of it is a mild intoxicant. The international literature is on the whole agreed that even long-term moderate use has not been shown to have serious ill effects. However, there are a number of problems, and we should be cautious about too optimistic a judgement on cannabis. One fact of importance is that there is enormous variation between samples of the drug: one analysis of cannabis 'joints' showed that the difference between the weakest and the strongest was 30,000 per cent! Another factor to bear in mind is that most of the sophisticated research on cannabis has taken place *since* 1972, and therefore one should approach some of the earlier studies with some degree of caution.

While it is fair to say that most of the dramatic warnings about the dangers of cannabis in the past have been shown to be ill-founded, there are certain dangers which should not be discounted, and these can be listed as follows:

1   The main active chemical in cannabis is a substance called delta-9-trans-tetrahydrocannabinol (THC). In recent years more work has been done on THC, and much of the cannabis in circulation contains a higher THC content than was the case before

the 1970s. In addition, THC itself may be in circulation (though much of what is called THC on the street market is actually other, more dangerous, drugs) as is 'hash oil' which may contain between 30 and 90 per cent THC. The high THC content alters our judgement on the effects of cannabis for these are related to potency, and there is no doubt that THC is a very powerful chemical indeed. A big enough dose can certainly produce a brief psychosis.

2   While cannabis is often compared, favourably, to alcohol, there is one important distinction. Alcohol is water-soluble, and its effects are washed out quickly from the body. Cannabis, however, accumulates in the body fat, and so the THC level will build up.

3   There are some studies, although the research is far from clear yet, which suggest that there may be harmful physical effects in connection with respiration and heart conditions.

4   It has been claimed that long-term use of cannabis can lead to a state of cumulative lethargy and loss of interest in life and activity. This condition has been called the 'amotivational syndrome', and some of those most favourable to the drug regard it as a worrying factor. However, the existence of the syndrome has been questioned, and one should not build too much upon it.

Many of the dangers attributed to cannabis are not proven, but it would be silly to ignore them simply because propagandists against the drug have overstated their case. However, there is one danger in cannabis use which has a lot of evidence to support its truth — the danger of imprisonment. While magistrates are less likely today to send first offenders to prison, there is still the danger that, through the operation of the drug laws or through police activity, cannabis users may be drawn into criminal groups. That is not an argument against the drug, but it needs to

27

be remembered as a fact of life in a country where 80 per cent of all drug offences are for cannabis, most of them being for simple possession.

Nobody knows the extent of cannabis use in Britain. A survey in 1969 suggested a million users, and another survey in 1973 claimed nearly four million. Between three and five million is possible. While the drug has replaced alcohol as a recreational agent in some circles, the evidence seems to suggest that, on the whole, it has rather been added to the range of drugs. It is also possible that many people have given up their use of it either on financial grounds or as a result of disappointment that the exaggerated claims for it were not fulfilled. Others, disappointed at the mild effects of cannabis *as smoked*, may be persuaded to try stronger forms, such as hash oil or synthetic THC (real or imagined) or to move on to more potent drugs altogether. However, while claims are often made that THC is in circulation in Britain, the evidence that this is so is far from conclusive.

3 LSD and the psychedelic drugs

The word 'psychedelic' was first used by a British physician in 1957 to describe drugs which enrich the mind and enlarge the vision. While the word was new, as were some of the drugs about which it was used, the use of drugs to enrich and expand consciousness, to open up new horizons, to increase creativity, and so on, is of great antiquity. The peyote cactus and a variety of sacred mushrooms have been used for spiritual purposes from early times. But the discovery and subsequent spread of lysergic acid diethylamide (LSD-25) introduced a new era in the use of drugs for such purposes.

LSD is derived from ergot, a fungus which grows on rye. It was discovered in 1938, but it was only in 1943 that its effects on the mind were recognized. In the early 1950s it was used in psychiatry, and a certain amount of therapeutic use of the drug continued down to the end of the 1960s. The value of the drug lay in its ability to open up areas of the unconscious quickly, and so to penetrate into buried experiences and emotions in very early childhood. There are two important effects of the drug which are crucial to understanding its popularity later in the psychedelic drug culture of the 60s. The first is its ability to reduce the critical faculties, and therefore to open up different ways of looking at reality. The second is its alteration in the method of processing incoming data by the mind. So things which formerly seemed trivial assume unusual importance. LSD seems to trigger a kind of depth charge into the unconscious: the direction which it then takes probably depends more on the context than on the drug.

Although LSD had been in use since the 1950s, it was not until the hippy phenomenon which grew up in San Francisco in 1966 that the drug came to hold a major role among young people. Since those days interest in the drug has subsided but is now increasing again. Looking back at that period and the alarmist press coverage, it is striking how few young people really came to grief as a result of the drug. The main danger was not so much a direct result of the drug as of a panic reaction to it, the so-called 'bad trip'. As use of the drug developed, fewer bad trips were reported, as users learned how to control its use and understood its possible effects. There is now a very extensive literature on the use and dangers of LSD, and there are few recorded fatalities. The real difficulties have occurred when, as a result of their experiences with the drug, people (not all of them young) with considerable personal problems and with very limited awareness of themselves have been confronted with too much reality too quickly. For some, this has been an experience of disintegration and terror. They have, in the words of one experienced LSD counsellor, 'gotten lost in inner space'. Some of them have never come back. However, one has to remember that such inner fragmentation often occurs without the use of chemicals, and we call it psychosis or madness. The critical question is not about whether drugs were used or not, but whether the individual was able to integrate and make sense of his new and strange experiences, or whether they reduced him to fear and confusion.

There is little reliable evidence of serious physical damage from LSD although there have been reports of chromosome breaks and of brain damage from time to time. In an American study of 25,000 LSD experiences ('trips') under supervision it was found that there were only two suicides and eight psychotic episodes. In Britain, a study of 50,000 trips showed three suicides and twenty suicide attempts, with thirty-seven chronic psychoses, most of which were resolved in three months. However, as with other forms of drug use, the context is crucial. One experienced doctor claimed that the worst thing that can happen to a person on a bad LSD trip is that he gets taken to a casualty department where he is treated by an innocent and unsophisticated physician. The individual who does not know his or her inner world may find the use of LSD without preparation or proper setting an experience of sheer hell. At the street level, a variety of chemicals of varying purity and doubtful identity have been sold as LSD. Other street drugs have been proclaimed as better and more potent than LSD. These have included the notorious 'peace pill' or 'angel dust' PCP (phencyclidine hydrochloride) which can lead to severe psychotic states, as well as various hallucinogenic mushrooms. The psilocybin mushroom has been used for years and remains popular.

Recently, after some years of declining use, LSD has re-emerged as a 'street drug', particularly (but not only) among pop-festival goers. But there are two significant differences with the earlier situation. First, as with cannabis, the older association with a subculture and an ideology has evaporated. Today's users are far more diversified than were the 'hippies' of the post-1967 era. Secondly, with the disintegration of a subcultural identity, there has also been a loss of the peer group support, provided by the subculture, for 'bad trips' and for panic reactions by naive users in general. So there are now more cases of young 'poly drug' users, i.e. people who use many different drugs, who may combine alcohol, glue and LSD, largely for escapist or recreational reasons. There may, of course, be subcultural preferences — punk, mod, skinhead, and so on — but most young

30

people cannot be fitted in under these labels.

4   Hypnotics, sedatives and tranquillizers

Hypnotics are drugs which induce sleep. But they can be taken like alcohol, as intoxicants, and can also be used to potentiate the effects of such drugs as heroin. Until the 1960s the main hypnotic drugs were the barbiturates. During the first half of the 60s the numbers of prescriptions increased to around 17 million, while the suicide rate from these drugs quadrupled. Suicides and accidental deaths from barbiturates continued to increase until the end of the 60s. Between 1959 and 1974, over 27,000 people died in England and Wales from barbiturate poisoning. During this period the number of prescriptions for these drugs totalled 225 million. However, as a result of considerable pressure from groups working with addicts and within the medical profession itself, the prescribing of barbiturates has been curbed. While the earlier barbiturate addicts tended to be middle-aged and female, there has been an increase in the last decade of the practice of injecting barbiturates, and most of these users are young. Again, while the number of prescriptions for barbiturates fell in the 1970s, the average size of each prescription rose between 1971 and 1977. In this period, deaths by barbiturate poisoning increased per million prescriptions while the total number of prescriptions declined. A 1978 study showed that barbiturates were a cause of death in 53 per cent of all drug-related deaths in London. The mortality figures for England and Wales for 1978 show 712 deaths from barbiturates of which 415 were suicide and self-inflicted injury, and 144 deaths from alcohol and barbiturates combined.

There is, however, a more worrying factor in the reduction in barbiturate prescribing. One reason for this may well be the fact that pharmaceutical companies can make more money out of the newer benzodiazepines which have to a large extent replaced them. There has, for years, been a major problem among the middle-aged in the abuse of drugs such as Mogadon, Valium and

Librium. However, in recent years, as barbiturates have declined, and the non-barbiturate drug Mandrax (methaqualone) once very popular with young users, has ceased to be manufactured in Britain, young people have turned to the benzodiazepines. Experience in one London surgery, in an area with a long tradition of adolescent drug abuse, has shown an increased demand for such drugs as Dalmane (flurazepam) and Ativan (lorazepam).

5 Opiates

Heroin

There is a legend that the opium poppy first grew on the spot where Buddha's eyelids fell when he cut them off to prevent himself from falling asleep. But opium had been mentioned long before this, and ancient writers were aware of its medicinal value. Opium abuse on a large scale developed in the seventeenth century, and it was during this century that preparations such as laudanum and 'Dover's Powder' were produced in Britain. A short course of withdrawal treatment for opium addiction was described at the end of the seventeenth century. It was in 1830 that morphine, which is a natural alkaloid of opium, was extracted, and it was followed a few years later by codeine. It was in the nineteenth century also that the hypodermic syringe, which has played such a crucial role in addiction, was invented by Pravaz. By the 1860s there was writing on the abuse of morphine, and by the 1880s the use of morphine and cocaine together was reported. In the 1890s heroin, a synthetic drug produced by heating morphine over acetic anhydride, was first produced. Most of these drugs (apart from cocaine) are derived from opium, and are therefore know as opiates.

In Britain, unlike the United States, it has been possible for many years for people addicted to these drugs to obtain them on medical prescription. This is sometimes known by the misleading term 'the British system'. In fact there never was an actual system

TABLE 3

Drug addicts known to the Home Office at 31 December 1973-81

Age	1973	1974	1975	1976	1977	1978	1979	1980	1981
0-19	84	64	39	18	21	36	34	34	84
20-24	751	693	562	412	389	438	428	396	629
25-29	530	684	756	809	825	945	1016	982	1232
30-34	134	163	219	250	357	511	672	852	1185
35-49	136	165	171	189	209	255	288	326	439
50+	180	196	194	189	201	205	206	209	216
Not recorded	1	2	8	7	14	12	22	47	63
All ages									
Females	446	509	511	487	550	696	774	837	1112
Males	1370	1458	1438	1387	1466	1706	1892	2009	2732
TOTAL	**1816**	**1967**	**1949**	**1874**	**2016**	**2402**	**2666**	**2846**	**3844**

Source: *Home Office Statistical Bulletin*, 29 June 1982

TABLE 4

Narcotic addicts not previously known to the Home Office notified during the years 1973-81

Type of drug taken at notification	1973	1974	1975	1976	1977	1978	1979	1980	1981
Heroin	509	525	524	606	614	860	1117	1151	1660
Methadone	147	165	156	140	170	159	182	152	207
Other drugs	151	182	242	238	324	333	315	297	381*
TOTAL	**807**	**872**	**922**	**984**	**1108**	**1352**	**1614**	**1600**	**2248**

*includes 244 notified as addicted to dipipanone

33

for dealing with heroin addiction because it was not felt in the early years of the drug's use that there was any serious problem. Addicts were few, and were all therapeutic addicts, that is, addicts who had been given the drug for the treatment of some condition, and had become addicted to it. In 1926 the Rolleston Committee recommended that it should be regarded as a legitimate exercise of medical responsibility to prescribe morphine, heroin and cocaine for addicts if treatment methods had failed and if there seemed a likelihood that they could function on a maintenance dosage of the drug. It is from this period that the so-called British system developed, and until the 1960s it seemed to be working well. In fact between 1935 and 1953 the total numbers of addicts fell from 700 to 290. They were mainly middle-aged and were addicted to morphine and other synthetic drugs. Only a small number were using heroin. There did not seem therefore to be any serious problem.

In 1961 another government committee reported on drug addiction in Britain. It concluded that there was still no cause to fear that any increase was occurring. In fact the Home Office figures show an increase from 1954 onwards, though in 1960 there was a slight fall, to be followed by epidemic increases from then onwards. But the proportions using heroin increased dramatically throught this period, and, unlike the earlier addicts, the new addicts were aged between 15 and 35. The first addict under the age of 20 appeared on the Home Office's list in 1960, and by 1968 there were 764. These, of course, are very small figures in relation to the general population. What caused alarm was not the overall size of the addict population, but its rate of increase. The figures showed a classic epidemic pattern. Moreover, unlike the older addicts, the new addicts almost all began to use heroin illegally, and none of them were therapeutic addicts. However, there was no evidence at this time of illegal heroin even though the heroin was being used by persons other than those for whom it was prescribed. All the heroin in circulation had come from chemists' shops on prescription for somebody. So controversy arose over the complicated question of 'overprescribing', an issue which is still a problem. What was happening was that the majority of addicts were concentrating in Central London as patients of a small group of doctors, some of them receiving very large prescriptions. It was from the surplus of prescribed heroin that the newer addicts came, and it is possible to show, on a chart, how the increase occurred. In 1968 the prescribing of heroin and cocaine for addicts was restricted to certain licensed doctors, and notification of addicts became compulsory.

It is worth pointing out at this point that, contrary to general opinion, there has never been such a thing in Britain as a 'registered addict'. From early days the Home Office kept a list, which was built up from notifications by doctors, and from checks at pharmacies (where dangerous drugs had to be entered in a special register). By this method, most addicts came to notice sooner or later. They did not register with anybody, except with their GP in the way anyone does. The correct term for them was 'known addicts'. In 1968 notification by doctors became compulsory, but it is still incorrect to speak of a 'registered addict'. One cannot register as an addict! It is also worth pointing out that the Home Office figures are much more reliable than is often claimed, but one has to understand their limitations. They have never claimed to include all known drug abusers, but simply to list, as fully as possible, all known addicts. Since almost all addicts became known, sooner or later, through doctors, chemists or police action, the figures until the late 60s were a reasonable guide. As the black market has increased since then, far more addicts who have derived their drugs entirely from unknown sources have appeared, and the official figures are less of a guide than they once were.

The increase in the black market in heroin has certainly been the most marked and most alarming feature of the history of the drug during the 1970s. One of the fears often expressed before the tightening up on prescribing occurred after 1968 was that such action would open the way for the black market to develop. The history of heroin addiction in the USA, where heroin had been banned for many years, was not encouraging. Heroin distribution was controlled by the Mafia, while in Britain the addict got his supply on a prescription from his doctor. The Mafia would move in if the source from overprescribing doctors dried up, it was claimed. Although the term 'Mafia' is often used as a synonym for 'criminal syndicate', it should be remembered that many different gangs are involved all over the world. Even in the USA the Mafia is only one criminal syndicate and probably not even the most ruthless as the Florida 'cocaine wars' showed. Some of the doctors themselves warned that this was already happening. As early as 1966 one doctor, with a large number of heroin addict patients, wrote:

> The most threatening portent is that addicts are telling me that there is plenty of the stuff to be had on the black market, even though the source from over-prescribing doctors is drying up. It looks as if big business, which has been waiting in the wings for so long, has now taken over the stage and is playing the lead.

The following year there were reports of powder heroin, that is illegally manufactured material. But it was not from the Mafia that the new wave of black market heroin came, but from the Hong Kong Triads, the well-established Chinese criminal syndicates. So, as doctors at clinics, which had been set up in the aftermath of the new legislation, began to substitute the long-acting drug methadone (Physeptone) for heroin, 'Chinese heroin' began to circulate on an increasing scale, first in London and then in other districts. By the mid-70s Amsterdam had become the centre for the organized traffic of the Triads. However, by 1979 the Middle East was taking over as a centre for illicit heroin, and Iranian heroin, which is refined directly from opium without a morphine base, was appearing in Britain.

It is impossible here to describe the complex developments within the world of the heroin addict, and the changes which have occurred since the late 60s. But several points are important. While there is evidence that the rate of increase of young addicts has slowed down, it would be a mistake to think that all is well.

It is claimed that the danger of the casual young teenage drug-user getting involved with heroin addiction is much less than it was, though evidence from various parts of Britain calls this into question. Within the heroin scene itself, the pattern has become much more criminalized, more dangerous, and (for the dealers) more financially lucrative. Illegal heroin means impure heroin, and so the danger of death from alien substances has increased. The increased involvement of the organized international gangs has meant more violence than was the case in the 60s. And there is evidence that, within certain circles, heroin addiction is increasing again. There is much talk of Britain having 'contained' the problem, but this is less than a half truth. Some clinics tend to see the original 1960s addicts who are simply getting older: they are 'containing' their addiction, rather than 'curing' it. But it would be wrong to conclude that all possibility of spread had been eliminated. The clinics have not 'contained' addiction as such, or even their own patients, who continue to obtain black market drugs. The situation is in many respects worse today than it was ten years ago.

There is still a good deal of confusion about heroin. In itself, it is a far less dangerous drug than many which attract less attention. It is, of course, highly and quickly addictive, but there would be relatively little to worry about if the only problem were heroin in isolation. Given the undesirability of people being physically addicted to anything, the management of heroin use does not present insuperable problems. The really serious problems are more connected with the life-style of the street addict, the social context in which the drug circulates, and the other drugs which are used alongside heroin. It is the opinion of many people that the needle and the needle culture are far more dangerous than the actual drug injected. Getting addicts off the needle is far more difficult than getting them off a particular drug. It is the needle which marks a real line of demarcation.

Although we have concentrated on heroin, it should be remembered that, with intravenous use, there is usually a variety of drugs involved. Few addicts use heroin alone, and so we must take into account drugs such as methadone, cocaine, barbiturates, and so on. In 1968 there was an epidemic of intravenous Methedrine abuse, and this was followed by the increased use of barbiturates by injection. This type of drug abuse has continued, and has led to very serious physical problems among street addicts.

However, injecting has never been a form of drug abuse favoured by more than a minority of the population. This is sometimes, understandably, received with relief by parents who feel that the disagreeable nature of the needle provides an effective barrier to their own children's involvement with dangerous substances. The recent upsurge in the popularity of *sniffing* heroin must therefore be viewed with concern and has to some extent broken down the barrier of the needle, thus allowing more casual, and younger, users to become involved. There are now far more 'suburban junkies' as well as many more young users of heroin and other opiates in areas of Britain which were not affected to a great extent in the 60s explosion. Thus, schoolchildren in Strathclyde accounted for a large proportion of 1,000 opiate users identified in a recent report by Glasgow University. The researcher claimed an increase of 500 per cent in the use of opiates in the area. This includes synthetic opiates such as diconal and palfium which are becoming extremely popular.

A major factor here is finance. It is ironical that in an inflationary period when the prices of most consumer goods, and of legal drugs such as alcohol, have risen steeply, one of the few things to have fallen in price in recent years is heroin. In 1981 around 800 kilogrammes was smuggled into Britain, and prices have fallen from £80 to £100 per gram to around £60 or even £40. Advice agencies are reporting an increase in inquiries from, or about, casual, first-time users, often being introduced to the drug at suburban parties.

6   Glue sniffing and solvent and abuse

One of the important lessons which has been learnt through the experience of recent years has been the fact that, when certain drugs are withdrawn from circulation or cease to be available, others take their place. Common medicines and products used in the home may become 'problem' substances. In recent years there has been much concern about the increase in 'glue sniffing' among young teenagers. Strictly speaking, the problem is not one of glue but rather of the use of vapours from a variety of products. Nor is it always sniffing, but also inhaling by mouth. There had been cases of the abuse of laughing gas, ethyl ether and chloroform in the nineteenth century, but the first reports of the new style of what is more precisely described as solvent abuse in Britain occurred in 1962. There had, however, been an epidemic in the United States in the late 50s beginning in California, spreading to the Mid-west by the early 60s, and to the East Coast by the middle 60s. In Canada too there was an increase in the abuse of glue towards the end of the 60s.

A whole range of products can be used, but they fall into three main categories: volatile solvents, aerosols and anaesthetics. Among solvents, the main substances which have caused concern have been toluene (a constituent of Evostick, Araldite, and other products), benzene (found in petrol and rubber solution), acetone, and the fluorocarbon propellants in aerosols. Products such as plastic model cements, household cements, nail polish remover, paint thinners, lighter fuel, cleaning fluids are among those used. Aerosols such as hair sprays, deodorants and insecticides are less common, but cases of abuse are found from time to time. Anaesthetics such as nitrous oxide, ether and chloroform, common in the nineteenth century, are still abused in the twentieth.

The method which young people use is usually to put a plastic bag with its open end against the nose and mouth. An alternative method is to use a handkerchief or rag soaked in the substance. The fumes are rapidly absorbed into the bloodstream, leading to

TABLE 5

Persons found guilty of, or cautioned for, drugs offences UK 1973-81

TYPE OF DRUG	1973	1974	1975	1976	1977	1978	1979	1980	1981
All drugs	14977	12532	11846	12754	12907	13604	14339	17158	17921
Cocaine	181	375	379	327	309	348	331	476	566
Heroin	435	444	393	464	393	483	520	751	808
Methadone	347	464	484	416	347	369	298	363	445
Dipipanone	198	369	409	361	378	493	453	440	498
LSD	1323	905	826	647	279	291	208	246	345
Cannabis	11476	9517	8987	9946	10607	11572	12409	14910	15388
Amphetamines	1777	1482	1501	1909	1788	1093	760	827	1074
Other drugs	1672	1654	1642	1293	1298	1262	1165	1292	1141

1   As the same person may be found guilty of or cautioned for offences involving more than one drug, rows cannot be added together to produce totals.

2   Includes offences under drugs legislation and other offences where drugs were also involved.

Source: *Home Office Statistical Bulletin*, 29 June 1982

a form of intoxication similar to alcohol. A third method is to use an aerosol spray and inhale. It is generally found that glue-sniffers are young males aged between 10 and 17, though in recent years more girls have come to notice. For the majority, it is a phase of adolescence and does not continue. There is no evidence to suggest that glue-sniffers are involved in any drug subculture, and the phenomenon is not connected with other forms of drug abuse. Often this type of abuse becomes a cheap way of getting drunk, and in many cases it is found among teenagers in run-down inner city districts.

As with all forms of drug use, some solvents are more harmful than others. Young people have died *directly* through sniffing butane gas and aerosols. But a serious danger is not from the glue or other substance, but rather from suffocation through the use of a plastic bag. Other dangers are that, as a result of the need to practise this form of abuse away from sight of adults, young people may choose dangerous places such as canal banks or buildings near busy traffic. Suffocation may also occur through inhaling of vomit while unconscious. While deaths are not common, there have been a number — 110 cases of death after sniffing had been reported in the USA by 1970 and cases were being reported in Britain. There have been claims of permanent brain damage based on a case in 1966, but this involved a man who had been sniffing a gallon of toluene every 4–6 weeks for 14 years!

A recent study of 140 deaths in the UK (1971–81) associated with volatile solvents showed that the median age was 16–18 years, and nearly 80 per cent were under 20. The male to female ratio was 13 to 1. Death rates were highest in the conurbations and in Scotland, Northern Ireland and Northern England. The chief substances used were butane, solvents in adhesives and other solvents, aerosols, and, in a few cases, fire-extinguishing agents. In about 49 per cent of these cases, death was attributed to the *direct* toxic effects of the substance.

For more detailed studies of these drugs, readers are referred to Appendix I.

Some recent changes

Finally, some points about other drugs and some of the changes which have occurred or seem to be occurring. Obviously, as new drugs are constantly appearing, it is impossible to predict accurately what new forms of drug abuse may emerge. From time to time, certain types of drug seem to reach a 'crest' when abuse subsides, and it may then decline. Often drugs may go out of fashion for a time, and then come back. Alcohol, which was out of favour with many young people in the 60s, is now back with a vengeance. While many young people seem to have turned away from the use of the needle, and to have recognized its dangers to health and to life, there is another side to that picture. Many needle-users have moved into the area of 'poly-drug abuse', that is, the use of a wide variety of drugs, pure and impure, legal and illegal, by injection.

So the crushed contents of barbiturate capsules, illegally manufactured, amphetamine sulphate powder, and many other dangerous substances may form part of the needle culture. As the black market grows, so the danger of impurities in the drugs increases. In Amsterdam, a study of street heroin a few years ago showed that over 50 per cent contained strychnine. While there is evidence to show that many young people have turned away from drugs in favour of other roads to satisfaction — religion, political action, violence — drugs never go away, and, as in other fields, things which were unfashionable in one generation return in the next. We need therefore to learn from the experience, including the mistakes, of the past, for 'drug problems' are never entirely new.

3

What is Drug Addiction?

So far we have talked about drugs, drug misuse, drug abuse, drug addiction. But what do these terms mean, and how do they differ from each other? Although the word 'drugs' often has pejorative associations, in themselves drugs are neither good nor bad. It is wrong to see the *use* of drugs as bad in itself. Penicillin, antibiotics, aspirin, cough mixtures, insulin — all these are drugs. Drug use must be distinguished from drug misuse and drug abuse. I shall use drug misuse to mean the *intermittent* wrong application of a drug or drugs, and drug abuse to mean the *continuous* wrong application of a drug or drugs. The drug misuser uses a drug wrongly, sometimes by mistake or by accident. The drug abuser puts it to a bad and harmful use. The misuse of some drugs can bring about drug addiction or dependence. For example, common drugs like the major tranquillizers (phenothiazines) and the minor tranquillizers (such as Librium and Valium) can bring about dependence, though these drugs do not, on the whole, figure in adolescent drug scenes.

So what is drug dependence and drug addiction? Nowadays official statements such as those from the World Health Organization tend to prefer the term 'dependence to addiction, and to distinguish the different types of dependence which vary according to the drug used. An earlier definition from the WHO issued in 1957 gave five characteristics of addiction, and, while they are not all found in every form of dependence on a drug, they are a useful starting point. Addiction usually involves:

1   an overpowering desire or need to continue taking the drug and to obtain it by any means;

2   a tendency to increase the dose;

3   a psychological and usually physical dependence on the effects of the drug;

43

4   the appearance of an 'abstinence syndrome', with symptoms of acute distress when the drug is withdrawn;

5   detrimental effects both on the individual and society.

In later definitions, the variation in types of dependence was stressed but the above characteristics are still applicable to the drugs with which we shall be concerned in this chapter. For simplicity, we shall use the terms 'addiction' and 'addict' rather than 'dependence' and 'drug dependent person'. By addiction, we shall refer to that type of dependence on a drug in which the above characteristics are present. Attention should particularly be drawn to the element of physical dependence, that is, the body comes to need the drug and suffers an 'abstinence syndrome' when the drug is withdrawn. Drug addiction is thus very different from casual experimentation. It is wrong to treat all drug abusers as addicts, or all drugs as equally addictive. Not all drugs produce physical dependence, and in some the level of dependence is higher than in others.

Also it is very important to remember that addiction is not simply a static property which exists within a drug and then attaches itself to a person. Addiction is a process which involves a number of forces — pharmacological, social, psychological, and so on. A relationship is created between a particular personality, with all that has gone to make up that personality, and the drug of his/her choice: and this relationship takes place within a specific social and cultural setting at a specific time in history. So many factors go to produce the drug addict: that person's own early history and family background; the properties of the chosen drug; the degree of availability of a drug in a given area at a particular time; and so on.

Until the last two decades, there were broadly two types of drug addiction which were common in Britain. The first involved people addicted to such drugs as morphine, heroin and pethidine, powerful pain-killing (or analgesic) drugs. The second consisted of people addicted to sleeping pills of barbiturate type. Both these types of addict were known as therapeutic addicts.

Sometimes their addiction is said to be 'iatrogenic', literally 'doctor-induced'. While such addiction is by no means extinct, the majority of young people have not started on their drug career in this way. However, it is essential to be aware of this pattern, since medical treatment, and proximity to drugs through working in a hospital, are important elements in the growth of addiction in many people. Many doctors and nurses have become addicted in this way. Take the case of Connie.

Connie is now in her 60s and had a happy childhood. She has never married and lived with her mother. In her late twenties Connie went into nursing. She had suffered from a number of physical illnesses which caused her to experience severe pain, and she was put on pethidine, a powerful pain-killer, in hospital. The next ten years saw her in hospital regularly with considerable pain, including low back pain. She was prescribed a variety of analgesics including DF 118 and methadone. She is still receiving methadone in oral form. Connie is heavily addicted, but she has never injected drugs, has no contact with any drug culture or with other addicts, and is a very conservative lady with conventional attitudes on most social and moral questions (including drug addiction!)

Or take the case of Mary.

Mary is a manic-depressive of middle age. She moves between periods of intense activity and periods of deep depression. Like Connie, she suffers severely from low back pain for which she has had operations. She has also been a patient in a mental hospital. She too was treated with pethidine, and several years afterwards this was changed to methadone. Her dosage has remained unchanged, and she carries on with her housework and other jobs. When she is well, she has voluntarily reduced the dosage for periods. However, when the drug was withdrawn altogether, when she was an in-patient at a mental hospital, a serious nervous condition followed.

Both Connie and Mary are physically dependent on, addicted to, their drug. But, unlike many young drug addicts, they do not inject, and they are not part of any drug culture or drug-taking community. Since the 1960s there has been a marked growth in the numbers of young people who have started to inject drugs through contacts made on the street market, and have later registered with doctors in order to maintain their source of regular supplies. For them, the needle is of the greatest importance. After injection, the addict feels a sense of peace and well-being. So *Frankie*, a young addict, describes her first experience of heroin.

The H. Oh my God, such heaven. Yet at first I was only elated. Pleasure. Then one day more than one jack, and I got high, so high. Oh, wonderful. I hope I never forget, and that I can remember that heaven. Because it is my life. And possibly my death. But I don't care. If I could die that way I'd be happy.

Physical addiction follows very quickly after the use of pure heroin, although it is not correct to say, as some do, that it is instantaneous. Time is needed for the chemical process of dependency to build up. For some individuals, however, the time may be quite short, only a few weeks. Not all drug takers are attracted by heroin or by the needle, and the fear that a very large percentage of the population might be in danger of becoming addicted is ill-founded. But for those who are drawn to heroin, the euphoria experienced is very powerful. Heroin kills both physical and emotional pain and brings peace. But the euphoria does not last, and, in order to maintain the effect of the drug, the dosage must be increased. If this is not possible, withdrawal symptoms will occur, and the addict is soon reduced to taking the drug entirely to avoid the terrors of withdrawal.

So the 'abstinence syndrome', or withdrawal symptoms, is of crucial significance in understanding addiction. With a drug such as heroin such symptoms can include yawning, rhinorrhoea (runny nose), tears, sweating, anorexia (loss of appetite) (mild symptoms); trembling, goose flesh, abdominal cramps, insomnia (moderate symptoms); restlessness, vomiting, diarrhoea, and weight loss (severe symptoms). The worst features of the abstinence syndrome can be controlled by the use of other drugs. To go through withdrawal without the aid of any drugs at all is called 'cold turkey'. The fear of the abstinence syndrome is perhaps the crucial feature of addiction: the pain of withdrawal, and pain associated with withdrawal, must be avoided at all costs. With drugs such as the barbiturates, the withdrawal process may involve dangerous fits.

So there is a physical basis for addiction. The drug becomes a part of the cell structure of the body. The addict needs the drug in order to be normal. But there are other factors. It is important not to overstate the purely physical dependence: the psychological dependence may be more important. What kinds of people are attracted by pain-killing drugs in the first place? What is the wider social context? Drug addiction is rarely accidental. Let us look then at five cases, none of them untypical, of young people who have taken the path of addiction.

Kate. Now in her 40s, she was an illegitimate child. No contact with either parent, and was placed in care. Early illnesses, especially asthma and bronchitis. Moved from her home in the north-west of England to London where she became a prostitute at the age of 18. This was in the early days of the pep pill epidemic, and she became heavily involved with Drinamyl, Dexedrine and other stimulant drugs, as well as with cannabis. Admitted several times to mental hospitals, she was there put on to anti-depressants. Several years later she had begun to use large amounts of barbiturates (Tuinal) on which she overdosed on a number of occasions. By the age of 30 she was heavily into heroin addiction and also injecting barbiturates and other drugs. She has had numerous 'cures' but always returned to drugs. Is now receiving methadone from a clinic, but uses heroin (black market) and a variety of other drugs. She lives for drugs which are her only way of coping with very deep sadness in her life.

Robert. In early 20s, from a middle-class family in the south-west of England. Was hospitalized at the age of three as a result of a squint, and spent some time in hospital as a child for various illnesses. At the age of 15 overdosed on Mandrax (hypnotic drug) and was admitted into hospital where he was identified as a potential drug addict. However, no help seemed to be available in his area, and within three years he was using morphine and barbiturates intravenously. He married at the age of 20 but the marriage broke up very quickly, and he returned to live with his parents. He was put into mental hospital under a compulsory order after he had set fire to his parents' home, and on discharge moved south to London where he became more heavily involved with black market heroin. Lives with a girl who is also addicted.

George. Late 20s. Comes from a broken home in a very run-down district of London with a very high delinquency rate. His mother married, for the second time, to George's father, but they separated when George was 9. He lived sometimes with mother, sometimes with father, and finally settled with mother, who, when George was 13, married a third time. While at school, George, and most of his friends, made regular appearances in the juvenile court; he truanted frequently, and was held to be below average intelligence. As a juvenile he had five court sentences, and at the age of 15 was sent to approved school. His younger brothers have also been before the court. At the age of 17 he began using heroin, getting his initial supplies from the surplus of another addict, and soon registering with a doctor in another part of London. Soon after this he was sent to borstal for possession of dangerous drugs, but on release quickly returned to the same doctor, and later to an out-patient clinic. Has worked intermittently, uses whatever additional drugs he can get, and has become more isolated from his former friends except those who are also addicted. Still lives in the same district where he grew up, and sees no hope of getting out.

Stella. In her mid-30s. Stella's mother died when she was very young, and she was brought up by her aunt, though the relationship with her father has remained strong. At the age of seven, she had rheumatic fever and was hospitalized for a long period. Her adolescence was difficult, she had a child at 16, and in her middle teens had begun to work as a prostitute. This entry into prostitution coincided with the peak of the pep pill period, and she was using 20 Drinamyl pills a day at the age of 17 when she was admitted into mental hospital. She spent time in hospital and prison, but at 19 was on 40 Drinamyl a day. Through her prostitution she developed a number of physical complications which were a cause of severe pain, and she was put on to strong analgesics. At the age of 23 she registered with a notorious doctor, who was later sent to prison, and was receiving large amounts of injectible Methedrine. At the same period she began to use heroin and other drugs by the needle route, and later registered with an out-patient clinic from which she received heroin and methadone. She has now ceased use of injectible drugs after a period as an in-patient, but is still a prostitute, and still heavily dependent on various oral drugs, particularly hypnotics and analgesics.

Philip. Youngest son of wealthy, upper middle-class parents. Mother active in church and social organizations and very busy, father a weak man who had moved into heavy drinking. Philip was sent away to prep school and public school. His relationship with both parents was poor since mother was absorbed in 'doing good' (including much help to other people's children) and father was away at work or exhausted. At 15 began to use cannabis and amphetamines, and later, at art school, moved on to heroin. It was only at this stage, after an arrest, that his parents became aware of his drug use. By this time, all relationship with them had broken down, he moved into a flat with his addict girlfriend, where, after several years, he overdosed and died.

These five examples could be multiplied into hundreds. As we look at the histories of these young people, certain common features stand out, although their social and family backgrounds are different in important ways.

First, there is some kind of family breakdown, not necessarily in the form of a 'broken' family, but certainly in a very basic breakdown of relationships between parents and child. By the time that adolescence arrives, a time, in all these cases, when drugs were accessible, the drug route seemed a way of distancing child from parents, and of 'solving' the apparently insoluble problems.

Secondly, in several of these examples, there is an early involvement with hospitals, or early experience of physical pain. Later comes the experience of mental and emotional pain to which powerful, pain-killing drugs seem an obvious solution.

Thirdly, there is an inability to establish relationships, especially sexual relationships. So prostitution, or relationships with other addicts, becomes the norm of human relations. So the addict is an isolated person, often with a low view of his or her self and potential.

Fourthly, it is important to note the chronology. In order to have a drug epidemic, three factors are necessary: the availability of the drug, a vulnerable population, and the means of bringing the two together. In all these cases, this was the case. So the dates and places were crucial.

Finally, we see how, in several cases, the life-style of the person comes to revolve entirely around the drug. The drug dominates all life and all activity: without it, the pain is unbearable.

There has been much discussion of the so-called 'pre-addictive personality'. But drug addicts cannot easily be fitted into the labelling processes of psychiatry. The most one can say is that the isolated, immature and inadequate individual appears most frequently among drug addicts. But what happened to such people before the production of heroin or later drugs? Clearly they are not unique to the second half of the twentieth century. We are talking then about certain personalities who, given the right conditions, are open to the possibility of becoming drug addicts, but who, in different circumstances, might 'solve' their problems by other methods.

What is certain is that, if one omits the 'therapeutic addicts', there are few cases of drug addicts whose history does not show very strong evidence of severe disturbance in personal and social life prior to their addiction. Addicts are often referred to as 'psychopaths', but such terminology can easily become no more than a form of labelling which tells us little. It is too easy to put such labels on people whose life-style and behaviour patterns differ from, or offend, one's own. At the same time, there is no evidence that opiates in themselves transform a 'normal', well-adjusted person into a disturbed psychopathic personality. It is more correct to say that certain personalities are more prone to become drug addicts than others. The immature, the hyper-sensitive, the isolated, passive person who cannot maintain stable relationships with others: these are obvious candidates for the addictive life-style. However, some authorities would reject the view which associates drug addiction with personality dis-order. The addict, they say, is one who has chosen the life-style, and may be a perfectly 'normal' person who has simply taken the drug for long enough to develop withdrawal symptoms.

The violent, anti-social psychopath does not seem, on the whole, to be attracted to heroin and the opiate drugs so much as to alcohol and the amphetamines. But certainly there are some heroin addicts who fit this description. Far more common is the immature, inadequate person who seeks immediate gratification for his needs, cannot easily cope with mood changes, and is aimless and purposeless in his general life and outlook. Unable to establish secure emotional relationships with people, he estab-lishes a deep relationship with the drug and the needle which often takes the place of sexual activity. But the love of the needle is also a form of self-destruction: the quest for release and free-dom becomes a form of slow suicide. The folk singer Bert Jansch expressed something of the heroin experience in his well-known song 'Needle of Death'.

Through ages man's desire
To free his mind, to release his very soul,
Has proved to all who live
That death itself is freedom for evermore.
And your troubled young life will make you turn
To a needle of death.

4

Why Do People Take Drugs?

As individuals, we are not isolated units in a social vacuum. We are all part of a culture and absorb its values, assumptions, norms, prejudices, and so on. Many of us resist and oppose elements in our culture, but we are influenced, to a very great extent, by the culture. To escape its influence requires considerable effort as well as personal courage. So most people conform to the standards of the prevailing culture. Minorities of 'rebels' or 'deviants' question these standards, or ignore them, or actively oppose them. Drugs are an integral part of mass culture, because we are a drug-using society, and the pharmaceutical industry is one of our major industries. So it is wrong to see drug-taking as such as a form of social protest: nothing could be more conventional and conformist than drug-taking.

However, groups may develop within a culture which propagate different and perhaps opposing values and norms from those espoused by the majority. It has become common to call sub-groups within a culture by the name of 'subcultures'; and to call groups which are actively opposed to the mainstream culture by the name of 'counter-cultures'. There are a number of drug subcultures which, for the drug-takers who belong to them provide information, social support and an identity. It is wrong, however, to speak of one drug subculture, for there are a number, and they are different. But it is equally wrong to neglect the way in which drug abuse and addiction may be a product, not of a subculture, but of the prevailing culture of a neighbourhood, a city, or even a nation. There are many places where the use of certain drugs is the norm rather than the exception. This often means that the rate of addiction is low because people are taught how to control their use of the drug. Often, however, abuse of a drug becomes endemic, built into life, within a culture. Take, for example, the abuse of alcohol in Scotland. A study in Glasgow has shown that 92 per cent of boys and 85 per cent of girls are drinkers by the age of 14. The problem of alcoholism among Irish Roman Catholics is a difficult and complex area: it has been suggested, by a Roman Catholic priest who has studied addiction, that 40−50 per cent of all addicts are Roman Catholics. To evaluate such a claim is extremely difficult, but it does point to the importance of culture, including religious culture, in the beginnings of addiction.

So, in asking *why* people take drugs, we need to take into account their social and cultural background, and the pressures upon them. A deprived neighbourhood, with bad housing, high delinquency rates, and unemployment, is an obviously vulnerable base for the growth of addiction. The ghetto districts of American cities, where heroin addiction and social deprivation often go together, are clear examples. There are many examples in British cities where addiction to alcohol and a wide range of other drugs is high within decayed inner-city districts. The environment makes a great deal of difference, though, of course, it is not the only factor.

A subculture, with its own newspapers, music, advice centres, and methods of communication, may provide a way in which some forms of drug use may spread, though it may also curb other forms. The hippy movement, which began in San Francisco in 1966 and spread to Britain the following year, was an important way in which the use of cannabis and LSD spread among those young people who identified with the movement. Through journals, through music, and through ordinary social contact, these drugs became part of the culture. But that same movement helped to curb the use of amphetamines and heroin as well as other drugs which it regarded as socially harmful.

Today the Rastafarian movement is an important force among black teenagers. It needs to be taken seriously and not dismissed as merely a form of anti-social behaviour or a passing trend. It is a spiritual movement of great significance for the future of black people in Britain. Within the culture of Rastafari, the use of cannabis, as an element within religious life, is important. Rastas use cannabis as the Native American Church has used peyote for many years, and as Christians have used wine in the sacrament. To treat such drug use as no more than criminal behaviour is to be insensitive almost to the point of total blindness.

Again, the kind of drugs which are available and acceptable within a country vary enormously. Guinness and whisky, not to mention the illegally distilled poteen, are acceptable in Ireland, where heroin addiction is very low. Heroin use is widespread in Hong Kong where cannabis is hardly used. In Jamaica, both cannabis and alcohol figure prominently in drug cultures. Between one-third and two-thirds of the lower class use cannabis. But there is no progression to heroin, which appears to be almost unknown.

Local cultures may also act not as promoters of drug use but as opponents of it. Take, for example, the low incidence of alcoholism among Jews. Jewish children are exposed early to alcohol within a religious context. Wine is consumed with meals, but excessive use is subject to disapproval. Or take the remarkable decline in heroin addiction in New York's Harlem since 1970, which seems to be due to a large extent to the strong disapproval within black families and the black community as a whole.

So young people may be drawn to drugs as a result of the approval, or lack of explicit disapproval, of drug use within their dominant culture. They may be dissuaded from drugs as a result of the strong disapproval expressed within their dominant culture. But they may also choose to discover through drugs experiences of which they feel the dominant culture has deprived them. Such experiences may be of recreation and pleasure, of release from pain, of deeper meaning in life, or simply of relaxation.

First, young people may choose to take drugs in order to experience intoxication, either within a social setting, or alone. Alcohol is the most common intoxicant. Most people drink socially, though the alcoholic, or the individual with a drinking problem will do so alone. Similarly, the young may use drugs such as cannabis or amphetamines or even glue as a way of 'getting high'. Glue-sniffing can be a cheap form of experiencing what adults obtain through alcohol.

Secondly, as we saw in the last chapter, some young people will turn to powerful pain-killing drugs such as heroin to kill emotional, rather than physical, pain. They seek release from an isolation and a degree of mental suffering which seems unbearable.

Thirdly, many young people may turn to drugs in order to find meaning in their lives. Drugs such as cannabis or LSD may seem to offer both an independence from the restrictions of adult society, and a sense of belonging. As the boundaries of ordinary experience are crossed, the drug user begins to experience a kind of transcendence of the kind which previous generations found through religion. So much modern religion seems to be based on convention and second-hand experience, and young people may seek a better, more vivid, more direct experience through drugs.

Fourthly, young people may take drugs, as adults do, simply in order to relax, to drift, to relieve the pressure, to slow down.

None of these experiences are new to us. All that is new is the type of drug which is used. Let's look now, in a little more detail, at what motivates many young people to use drugs in these ways.

Intoxicants

First, the use of drugs as intoxicants. To intoxicate oneself with drugs is well within the conformities of western culture. Alcohol as a social lubricant, an agent to facilitate discourse and conviviality, is widely accepted. The Psalmist speaks of 'wine that maketh glad the heart of man'. There is a world of difference between the use of alcohol in this social setting, and its use to drown sorrow. Today, however, many young people use cannabis as an alternative intoxicant to the majority drug, alcohol. Cannabis too is a social drug, not a solitary drug. It is used in order to 'get high' with friends. What do people seek by getting high? Precisely what human beings have always sought through the use of social intoxicants: a sense of ease in conversation; the ability to communicate within the group; increased enjoyment of music and dancing; the temporary removal of inhibitions; and so on. Often the shy, reserved person will use a drug in order to mix socially, to talk more freely. Cannabis is not unlike alcohol in its social use, and it is itself a mild intoxicant.

Amphetamines are also used in this way, although they are stimulants of the central nervous system; they increase activity rather than reduce it. Amphetamines may serve a dual purpose of enabling the person to stay awake for all-night parties or discos, and of enabling the shy person to overcome his shyness and embarrassment.

Many of the drugs which young people use to get high are actually depressants. Taken in large quantities they will bring about sleep. But if one then resists the sleep effect, one gets drunk. Alcohol, barbiturates, and other hypnotics, sedatives and tranquillizers are used in this way.

Many people come to no great harm, and may actually be helped in their social maturation, by the use of drugs as intoxicants. Thus the great social value of the English pub. On the other hand, among those who seek intoxication are some who cannot mix, cannot relate, cannot communicate without artificial aids; and for these, use of drugs can aid their growth into adult life, though continued reliance on them may retard that growth.

Pain Killers

Secondly, the use of drugs to kill, or avoid, pain. Pain can be mental and emotional as much as physical. It may be self-inflicted or self-imagined pain. Unlike the social drinker or cannabis user, the genuine addict is often a lonely, isolated person. He seeks more than escape: he seeks release from himself, the responsibilities of the world, his own inner suffering. This may lead him to excess use of the same drugs which others use as social intoxicants. Alcohol, for example, becomes for the alcoholic not a means to enhanced enjoyment of life, but a way of life in itself. Morphine and heroin act differently from alcohol, but both are narcotic, that is, sleep-producing. But the main medical use of these drugs is as analgesics, to kill or deaden pain.

To kill pain by drugs is not a strange thing to do. Society has taught us to do this. Pain is seen as bad, to be avoided at all cost. Whatever the trouble, there must be some chemical solution, some pill, which can be taken to deal with it. The inability of many people, not only young people, to experience pain, is itself a more dangerous phenomenon than the use of drugs, for it deadens and numbs the spirit. However, while heroin is used medically, as in terminal cancer, to kill pain, it does not follow that the young heroin addict has experienced overwhelming pain. In many cases it is the inability to develop even the emotional resources to deal with ordinary pain which has led them to heroin. Once addicted, it is the fear of the pain of withdrawal, often grossly over-dramatized, which keeps them on the drug.

Alcohol is also used by the heavy drinker to cope with pain. The solitary alcoholic will seek to 'drown his sorrows', to surround himself and his tragic existence with temporary oblivion, to block painful experiences. However, while there are similarities, there are often striking differences between the solitary drinker and the heroin user. The alcoholic, who is often of an older generation, has in many cases been through considerably more experiences in life than has the immature young junkie. There has often been broken marriage, wartime injuries, unemployment, a range of personal tragedies. Alcoholism is the result of a life marked by much suffering. Yet the alcohol does not kill the pain, it simply covers it for a while. The pain stays, and the alcoholic remains fundamentally a sad person, deeply broken, full of remorse. The young heroin addict is more likely to be an inadequate, childish individual, who has chosen to relate to a drug and a needle rather than to a person or persons. If the drug and the needle are removed, the relationship which needs to be built up with people invariably has to start at a level of childlike dependence.

To find a meaning in life

Thirdly, the use of drugs to find meaning in life. The obvious drugs which are used in this way are those of LSD type, the so-called 'psychedelics'. The word means 'mind-expanding'. Through the use of such drugs, the user seeks not to increase or decrease activity, not to block painful experiences, but rather to widen his horizons, to experience new aspects of reality. Because these drugs have not, on the whole, been favourites with adults, the use of them is one major way of asserting independence of, and creating a distance from, the adult world. It is part of the search for freedom from adult values and constraints. Irrespective of whatever the drug itself may do, its very status in the youth culture has had a major significance.

With the psychedelic drugs — LSD, mescalin, psilocybin, DMT, STP, PCP, and, to a lesser degree, cannabis — we are considering a class of chemicals which seem unique in their effects. To summarize them and the reasons for their use could occupy volumes, but we can refer to three important reasons. First, young people may use these drugs to increase self-knowledge. LSD was once referred to by over-optimistic psychiatrists as 'the royal road to the unconscious'. Through using it, people will seek to go into themselves at a deep level, to know themselves, to enter into their unconscious. They will hope, through this deeper awareness of self, to come back more whole, more aware, more honest people.

Linked with the quest for deeper awareness of oneself is the desire to move beyond the artificial boundaries of waking consciousness. Through LSD and similar drugs, it is hoped that the individual can transcend this consciousness, move beyond the ego, and perhaps achieve something of unity with the cosmos. People often describe this experience as one of 'cosmic consciousness' or 'expanded consciousness'. They may describe it in religious or mystical terms. Take the case of Raymond.

Raymond is a sensitive, artistic young man. His early life was very conventional, and his parents regular churchgoers. However, he felt that their religion was superficial and second-hand, and it did not seem to be based on any direct experience of God. After taking LSD he became deeply religious, identified his experience with that of the mystics and spiritual teachers of the East. He read the works of Alan Watts and Hermann Hesse, and came to believe that LSD was a breakthrough from modern materialism into the repressed, almost forgotten regions of the spirit which religious people talked about, but had not actually experienced for themselves. Raymond no longer takes LSD, but he does not regret his experience which he sees as a kind of conversion.

Raymond's experience points to a third aspect of LSD use — the desire to escape from the materialism and dreary convention of western society. Many young people who have used psychedelic drugs believe that our society, including its religious life, is deeply un-spiritual, indeed anti-spiritual. They believe that through LSD they can achieve a real spiritual breakthrough to deeper levels of consciousness, and so begin to see the meaning in human existence. Of course it would be ridiculous to imagine that all who use psychedelic drugs have these deep concerns: equally, it is irresponsible to ignore them as part of the total drug scene.

Relaxation

Finally, the use of drugs to relax. Many people young and old, use drugs not to get high in company with others, nor for any profound spiritual reason, nor to meet any deep emotional need, but simply to relax, to slow down, to reduce the pressure at the end of a heavy day. For many people under great pressure the tranquillizers, drugs such as Librium and Valium, are constant companions. For others the nightly glass of whisky is a favourite drug to help relaxation. Which drug is used will depend on many factors other than the properties of the drug. Certain drugs may be common and highly acceptable in one culture, but frowned on in another. Acceptable drugs change from time to time. Take, for example, the warnings issued by a distinguished Regius Professor of Physics at Cambridge at the turn of the century about a commonly used substance. It 'appeared to us to be especially efficient in producing nightmares with … hallucinations which may be alarming in their intensity'. Another quality of the same drug was 'to produce a strange and extreme degree of physical depression'. If the drug was taken at breakfast time, an hour or two afterwards 'a grievous sinking … may seize upon a sufferer, so that to speak is an effort…The speech may become weak and vague…By miseries such as these, the best years of life may be spoilt'. The drug to which the learned Professor was referring was the very English phenomenon, the cup of tea.

There are many other reasons why people take drugs: the influence of peers; sheer curiosity; the desire for new and strange experiences, especially those with an element of risk and danger; rebellion sometimes, desire to conform at others. The causes of drug use are almost as numerous as are drug users. But it is essential to re-emphasize how deeply entrenched drug-taking and drug abuse is in western culture. It would have been very odd indeed had there been no drug problem among the young. In fact, there is some evidence that young people may be turning away from the drug-abuse patterns of their parents.

The media

There are a number of aspects of the spread of drug abuse which need to be mentioned in conclusion. The first is the influence of the media. There is no doubt that irresponsible press coverage can actually produce a problem where previously there was none; and that fears which have no factual basis can be reinforced by the press. In 1972 the Consumers Union (USP) published an article called 'How to start a nationwide drug menace'. It recounted the story of the handling of some early cases of glue-sniffing. In the early 1960s there had been a number of reported deaths from glue. They were repeated over and over again although there was no clear evidence to show that any of them was definitely due to glue. One newspaper in Denver investigated reports of a few incidents of glue-sniffing in Arizona and

Colorado. They printed scare-type headlines combined with illustrations and instructions of 'how to do it'. The reports were followed up elsewhere. Within a few years a fairly minor problem had been manufactured into a national epidemic with mass-produced panic reactions, including probably an increase in glue-sniffing in dangerous places. The Consumers' Union study concluded:

> The effort to frighten people away from illicit drugs has publicized and thus popularized the drugs attacked. The impact on young eyes and ears of the constant drumming of drug news stories and anti-drug messages is clearly discernible — just look around.

In considering the reasons for drug-taking, the influence of press, radio and TV, pop stars, and so on should not be ignored.

Availability

A second important aspect is the question of availability. It is obvious that a drug epidemic will only occur if the drug is available. International politics can be directly relevant to the death of one teenager in a city street. For example, Alfred McCoy's disturbing book *The Politics of Heroin in South-East Asia* (Harper and Row, 1972) showed with considerable detail how American diplomats and secret agents were involved in the heroin traffic through alliances with groups involved, through covering up for known traffickers, and through active help in the transport of opium and heroin. Opium traffickers were, and are, supported as a military bulwark against communism. Both the CIA and its predecessor the OSS aided groups in Sicily and Marseilles who were the early importers. The OSS used Corsican syndicates to break up communist-led strikes. In the USA itself, when Robert Kennedy became Attorney-General, he found that 400 FBI agents were assigned in the New York City area to investigate communism, but only four to investigate the Mafia who were in control of virtually all the traffic in heroin.

Or again, since the late 1970s more heroin has been coming to Britain from Iran. The reason for this is that, under the Shah, there was strict control of opium production. Since 1979 the use of alcohol has been suppressed, but controls on other drugs have been relaxed, though the regime executes people on a regular basis for trafficking in heroin.

Of course, for those who are heavily addicted, a source for their drugs will always be found. But many drug-takers will be deterred from further use if the drug becomes difficult to obtain. This may involve action in places thousands of miles away from home. For the drug traffic is international.

Legislation

Availability raises the question of legislation. This is a complex area, and it is impossible to go into it in depth here. But it is important to stress that drug use may rise as a result of excessively strict legislation or of the opposite. Take, for instance, the history of the prohibition experiment in the USA. From 1920 alcohol was prohibited for beverage purposes. Between 1920 and 1924 the population of the federal prisons doubled, almost all of the new inmates being violators of the Volstead Act which had introduced prohibition. The trade in illegal liquor became a major industry. The cocktail became firmly established in American life as a way of making industrial alcohol drinkable. Organized crime became an integral part of American society during the prohibition era. The outlawing of heroin, which had occurred some six years earlier, paved the way for the Mafia which quickly took over control of addiction.

There is abundant evidence that attempts to stamp out addiction by repressive legislation may serve to drive it underground and thereby increase both the numbers of addicts and the dangerous nature of the drugs in circulation. The problem is to achieve a form of control which does not lead to more problems. Again, the question of the need of a drug in a given culture is important. During the early 1960s legally manufactured amphetamines were circulating in Central London in enormous quantities. An Act of 1964 gave the police power over possession, but nobody had any control over manufacture and distribution. It was only when the danger of amphetamines led to an increased reluctance of doctors to prescribe them that the amounts in circulation were reduced. Even now, the presence of one or two doctors who are willing to feed the illicit market can change the drug scene very quickly. Almost all the Methedrine in circulation in London in 1968 came from two surgeries.

So the prescribing habits of doctors, the manufacturing habits of drug companies, and the entry of a manufactured drug on to the street market are all key factors in whether certain drugs will be used or not. Even when the circulation of drugs such as amphetamines is curtailed, there are always some illicit laboratories. There is even illicitly manufactured Valium in the USA!

Ignorance

Finally, the effect of ignorance on drug use. Some people are opposed to the dissemination of drug facts on the grounds that this encourages drug abuse. So it may. However, one cannot prevent young people from experimenting with drugs, and it is best to ensure that the information they have is accurate. Many people come to grief through ignorance or through incorrect information. The unwillingness of many doctors to trust their patients with any information at all about the drugs prescribed for them has probably contributed both to the false mystique surrounding both the doctor and the drug, and indirectly to the spread of drug abuse. The spread of reliable drug information from credible sources is one of the best safeguards against drug-related harm.

5

Prevention, Treatment and After-care

To prevent young people from experimenting with drugs is simply not possible. When we use the word prevention, we are wiser to use it in its older meaning, derived from the Latin, of 'going before'. We need to try to discover the most constructive and sensible ways of preparing the way for children to grow up safely and behave wisely in a world where drugs will increasingly be available. To think in terms of panic measures, of sheltering young people from exposure to drugs, and so on is really to miss the mark. The best form of prevention is long-term care and support. The environment is so important here. We know that the great killer diseases have been reduced more by changes in the environment than by the use of medicines. Similarly, the most effective way of preventing harm from drugs is the creation of a safe, warm, loving atmosphere at home, in which communication is encouraged, in which the child's own worth and value are recognized, and in which support and help are always available.

In looking at the background of drug addicts and drug abusers, there are many different factors. Certain features do stand out with such frequency that they need to be stressed. Poor relations with parents, either because the family is broken, or because communication within the family has broken down, are a common feature, as is conflict within the family. The awareness that one or other parent seeks resolution of conflict through the use of alcohol or other drugs may encourage the child to follow in the parent's footsteps. There are many examples of young drug addicts whose family included one alcoholic or heavy drinker. Again, complete lack of discipline, or the opposite, ridiculous over-protectiveness or thoughtless discipline, are often present. So as parents we need to look to the factors in our own lives which are likely to lead to breakdown of relationships with our children.

Prevention

Three areas stand out as being of great importance in preventive work. First, the building up of a family environment in which affection is shared and expressed, in which young people are listened to and treated as important, in which parents take time to treat the concerns and problems of their children seriously, is of the greatest importance. In my experience and that of others who have worked with drug abusers, many come from homes where, while there is material security, there is no sense that the parents are able to spend time listening to their children, and so the comprehension gulf grows wider.

Secondly, the exercise of reasonable, firm but kindly discipline is necessary. Children need to know where they are. But disciplines and rules need to be explained, discussed and, if necessary, changed. Unreasonable discipline, which is based on nothing more than fear, prejudice or parents' un-thought-out assumptions is as useless as no discipline at all. Similarly parents who are continually changing their positions merely create an atmosphere of insecurity for their children. Discipline must be based on thought, respect for the child, and honesty.

Thirdly, parents need to take an honest look at their own drug problems, and their own use of drugs. Again, unreasonable attitudes, double standards, and the refusal to face these ambiguities, can create trouble for the future. Many alcoholics have come from homes where total abstinence was demanded from an early age, and where all alcohol was taboo. Parents who introduce their children to the social use of wine with meals, and who express disapproval of excess, are more likely to help them to a responsible approach to the use of this and other drugs.

However, while the family is of crucial importance in the formation of the young drug user, there are community aspects. It is important that parents are aware of, and in touch with the agencies and facilities in the local and wider community which are used by their children. Young people are affected to a considerable extent by the life-styles in their environment, and districts in which drug abuse is common play an important role in adolescence. The early epidemic of pep pills coincided with the era of the big discothèques, many of which were the first centres for distribution of the drugs. Often cafés and clubs are centres for drug dealing. In 1966, several youth workers in a very deprived area of London tried to identify certain types of youngster who were most at risk in relation to drug abuse. They identified three main types: the adolescent from a socially deprived neighbour-hood who leaves school at 15 and becomes a member of a highly delinquent and socially disorganized group; the totally alienated adolescent from the suburbs; and the adolescent who drifts into a large city and has no roots.

In relation to the first type, which was the group with which the workers were particularly concerned, they compiled a list of ab-out twenty young men and two girls who were felt to be in danger of becoming addicts. This prediction was based on the fact that they were delinquents, were regular users of certain cafés in the area, and were seen regularly in the company of known drug addicts. In all cases the prediction was 100 per cent correct. But the workers felt that, by this stage, effective prevention was impossible. They stressed the importance of working with a much younger age group, since the social causes had built up over a long period.

The youth and community worker is often in a strong position, in association with other agencies, to be of help to both children and parents. It is important for parents to accept that, on many questions as well as those associated with drugs, they are not the best people to be of direct help to their own children. In some areas, multi-disciplinary teams of youth workers, probation officers, physicians, and others have been able to share their experience and expertise and work together in the field of pre-ventive work.

The role of the school and of educational agencies is also of importance here. Nowadays, there is less concern in schools to teach specifically about the 'evils of drugs', and more concern to place 'drug education' in the wider context of health and social studies. Some of the earlier 'scare' teaching was counter-productive. It served both to encourage experimentation, and to reduce confidence in information from adult sources. Much of the literature aimed at teachers was quite unhelpful. One local education authority circulated a list of 'signs' of drug use for which teachers should watch out. All the signs were common signs of adolescent behaviour, and in one school, where the pupils found the list on the teacher's desk, they deliberately exhibited all the signs! Today, there is much better access to reliable information, and many schools have encouraged their pupils to do projects on drug use. However, scare tactics are not a thing of the past, as recent reaction to solvent abuse has shown. But again, it is essential to stress that education about drugs may not prevent experimenting. It may not increase it either. Its main aim is to reduce the level of harm.

Some parents who are also teachers are in direct contact with the educational task in relation to this and other areas of social studies. Others may be in positions where they can influence and help to educate those who frame or implement policy, those who can affect the future of the young drug taker for better or worse. Education about drugs is a matter of the 'long haul'. We need to set our sights on the long-term future, on trying to shape programmes, approaches and ways of looking at the issues which will pay off in the next generation. So the education of police, magistrates, clergy, social workers, and so on is a key area. Magistrates are in a very critical position, and there is a lot of evidence that harsh sentencing for minor drug offences in the past actually helped to increase the addict population. Lord Hailsham's wise words to magistrates in 1973 are worth remembering: 'My advice to you if you happen to come across the use of a soft drug is not to dive off the deep end. Take great care ascertaining the background, and treat the offender with becoming moderation.'

Preventive work is concerned with the reduction of harm, and this must include harm not only to the drug abuser but to his family and friends. This is an aspect of the question which is often neglected, and is of crucial importance. Parents of drug users need help too. Their reaction to the discovery that their son or daughter is using drugs may go through several stages. Shock and disbelief are common. 'It couldn't happen to my son.' Sometimes, a tragedy within a family, although painful, can be the only way of bringing parents to adopt more reasonable and compassionate attitudes. Sadly, there are many cases where the child is sacrificed, but the parent emerges a wiser and more caring person. There may be a sense of numbness and helplessness, and this may be followed by bitter resentment. 'After all we've done for you....' There may be a search for scapegoats — the bad company, the teachers, the doctor, and so on. There may be a rejection of the child.

Drug addiction is a family illness. It affects the entire family, not just the addicted member. In fact, it is often the parents, the brothers and sisters who need more help and support than the drug user. This can be a humbling and yet difficult experience, particularly for those parents who have often been of great help and guidance to other people's children, and now find themselves broken and helpless. There is a real danger now that such parents will put all the blame on themselves. So it is essential that, as a parent of a drug addict, you *seek help for yourself*. The appearance of drug addiction within a family can bring intolerable stress and pressure, and can lead to serious breakdowns within the family. If we are going to be of help and strength to others, we must ensure that we are receiving help and strength from others.

Often the shock of discovering that one's own child is using drugs brings about a necessary change in the attitude and approach of the parents. Listen to the words of a senior police officer whose son was found to be using heroin:

I had shared what I believe was the typical policeman's attitude — that drugs were a form of weakness or self-indulgence justified by any social or political excuse from rebellion or war to hatred of the capitalist system and I shared the view that it should be firmly stamped on. I now learnt that fighting the drug taker doesn't work. The deeper problems involved usually can be met only with understanding, and the parent is often best suited to be a kind of sheet anchor.

Understanding and love must go together and support each other. It is not helpful for the parent to assume all responsibility, to allow the child to evade all responsibility for his actions, to prevent him from suffering. Compassion means 'suffering with': if there is no suffering, there can be no compassion.

Emergencies

The treatment of drug addiction is not a simple matter. There are many different approaches, some of which work for some people, others for others. It is a question of 'different strokes for different folks'. But all drug abuse involves crises from time to time and often these need hospitalization. The commonest is overdose, and the parents may be in a position of having to 'bandage up' their drug-using child. The treatment of drug poisoning and overdose is a medical matter, but certain basic guidelines are important to know.

1   In cases of overdose, don't move the patient unless it is absolutely necessary. Place face downwards with head turned to one side. Do not prop up in a chair, or allow the person to lie on his back.

2   Loosen any tight clothing. Keep all airways clear. Check breathing and raise the chin. If unconscious, try artificial respiration. Call an ambulance. (In London in particular, it may be quicker, in cases of mild overdose, to ring for a taxi.)

3   Try to identify the drugs used, and take them to hospital with you along with any packets and any vomited material.

4   If the overdose is the result of glue or vapours, remove the person from the contaminated area.

5   Verbal reassurance can be important even when the person is apparently unconscious.

6   In cases of 'bad trips' from LSD, verbal reassurance is the most important treatment. The 'talk-down' method is preferable to medication. Bring the person down gently, in a quiet room, with subducd lights. Avoid rapid or sudden movements, and quietly reassure the person that he is still himself. The amphetamine psychosis ('the horrors') cannot be dealt with in the same way, and will need medication, verbal reassurance will help to control the person in the meantime.

The treatment of drug poisoning in hospital varies with the drug used. Amphetamine is readily absorbed from the gastrointestinal tract but less readily from the nasal and buccal (mouth) mucosa. Urinary excretion begins within about three hours of an oral dose, and nearly half the dose has usually appeared within 48 hours. Treatment is usually by gastric lavage, and phenobarbitone will probably be used. Barbiturates also are readily absorbed from the stomach and rectum, but complete excretion of long-acting compounds may take a week. With phenobarbitone poisoning, there may be prolonged coma and respiratory complications. Treatment will then involve the giving of oxygen and restoration of the blood pressure, and amphetamine may be used. With methaqualone (Mandrax) poisoning, the treatment will be intensive supporting therapy without forced diuresis.

It is important that people without medical knowledge do not use drugs in treating overdose instead of calling for an ambulance. In fact, inactivity is often the most positive treatment in non-fatal cases. No drug can restore uncomplicated, normal functioning faster than healthy inactivity and excretion. In the treatment of drug-induced psychoses, the drugs known as the phenothiazines are often helpful. But the treatment of overdose with medication does require specialized knowledge. There are many guidebooks on this area which, while they are intended for medical personnel, contain useful information for parents and non-specialists. See, for example, Peter A. Czajka and James P. Duffy, *Poisoning Emergencies* (The C.V. Mosby Company, St Louis, Toronto, and London, 1980).

Out-patient treatment

There are a number of out-patient clinics located throughout the country. They vary both in their quality of care and in the scope of their concern. Many of those which were set up after the 1968 legislation only deal with addicts of heroin and related drugs. They are concerned with maintenance more than with cure and, with the increase in new addicts, often less with maintenance than with 'cut-down' prescriptions. Addicts who register with a clinic will probably be taken off heroin and put on to a programme of oral methadone, in tablet or linctus form. This is known as 'methadone maintenance', a form of treatment which uses one drug to act against another. Methadone is a long-acting synthetic drug, and it has a twofold value. First, it takes people off the needle and the short-acting opiates. Secondly, it enables those using it to maintain themselves in employment, though this can be exaggerated. Those who promote methadone maintenance would not deny that they are replacing one addictive drug by another. But they would point out that wholly drug-free programmes only appeal to about 10 per cent of addicts, while methadone is acceptable to upwards of 60 per cent. Experience in a number of British clinics shows that methadone patients hold down jobs, and the crime involvement is not high. However, this is not a cure for addiction so much as a method of control and containment. It is an acceptance of the idea that often, and for periods of time, one should opt for limited goals. This applies also to those injecting drugs: clean needles, the use of disposable equipment, avoiding sharing needles, keeping one's skin clean, are all important as ways of preserving life and health.

Other kinds of out-patient clinic are the psychiatric clinics which deal with adolescent problems generally. These can be more helpful, for often the worst thing one can do with a young person using drugs is to label him as a 'drug problem'. Drug use may only be the surface feature, not the most important thing at all. The immediate contact person will in many cases be the GP. Even though he may not feel able to deal with the problem personally, it is often easier for him to make the referral to the clinic. At a clinic, the psychiatric social worker is normally the person who sees the patient first, and may then maintain contact with the family.

The out-patient clinic may thus be a place for the maintenance of an addict by providing him with regular supplies of drugs, or it may be a place where the young person experimenting with drugs may be helped to understand and cope with his own personal problems and needs. It is important to find out the kind of facilities which exist in a particular area.

In-patient treatment

Addicts may be admitted into hospital after overdose, or under a compulsory order, or through a request for withdrawal. Many addicts are withdrawn in the hospital wings of prisons. Again, in-patient units vary a great deal. Some, because of their facilities and the location in which they are set, can be no more than cleaning-up stations to which the addict can come for withdrawal and general overhaul, and from which he can return to the drug scene. Others can be more thorough and can attempt the beginnings of a process of treatment which will include after-care. But while dealing with the addict in the acute stages of drug intoxication or withdrawal is relatively simple, many addicts drop out of the long-term treatment programme because it makes too many demands on them.

In fact, hospital is unlikely to be a suitable place for the long-term treatment, which demands resources which are not purely medical and clinical, but which treat the drug user as a whole person and pay attention to his need to build up a new life-style.

Therapeutic communities

For this reason, the best hope for long-term change is the therapeutic community which is concerned to see drug abuse in a wider context. Again, there are many different types working in the field. Some operate at a street level, and offer basic medical and social care and perhaps accommodation to the using addict, with the possibility of referral to a residential community after withdrawal. Others accept a person only when he is withdrawn from drugs, and make considerable demands upon him. They may reject the 'professional' approach which sees the addict as a 'problem' to be 'dealt with' by experts. Instead they will see the addict as a person who needs to take initiative and accept control over his own life. One house which lays the emphasis on conscious effort includes the following passage as a daily morning reading.

> We are here because there is no refuge finally from ourselves. Until a person confronts himself in the minds and hearts of others, he is running. Until he suffers them to share his secrets, he has no safety from them. Afraid to be known, he can know neither himself nor any other — he will be alone. Where else but in our common ground can we find such a mirror? Here, together, a person can at last appear clearly to himself, not as the giant of his dreams, or the dwarf of his fears, but as a man — part of a whole, with his share in its purpose. In this ground we can each take root and grow, not alone any more as in death, but alive to ourselves and to others.

Some therapeutic communities are motivated by a Christian or other spiritual basis. Others, such as Synanon and Phoenix in the USA, are not religious, although their structure in many respects resembles a kind of secular monastery. Most of them stress the need to create a wholly new life-style, a drug-free environment and a new set of values and life objectives. When a person is heavily addicted, it is often the case that only a radical transformation of this kind can effect real change. Anything less is simply tinkering and is likely to fail. It is therefore particularly sad that, as a result of the economic situation and government policies, some valuable work is likely to collapse. For example, two Christian centres for after-care of addicts closed in May 1981, representing a loss of fifty beds.

However, as we stressed earlier, not all drug abusers are addicted to this degree. Many simply 'mature out' of addiction as they themselves grow up. Others fall in love, and the greater relationship makes the lesser one obsolete. For many, hospital and the clinic play an important role. But the addict is rarely 'cured' by medical care alone, for addiction is not a purely medical matter. Hence the need, whether in preventive work, in treatment or in after-care, to provide help and support for the individual within his social context. Within that context, parents have a role to play, but need always to remember that they are not the only people involved.

6

Some Practical Do's and Don'ts

In many respects, adult over-reaction to 'the drug problem' can be more harmful than the drugs themselves, and can make a difficult situation worse. It is necessary to remember that not all drug use raises serious problems. Much of it is purely recreational or experimental, and to make too much of it may be to build up into a major crisis what is in fact something quite small. So it is important not to panic, or to imagine that we can create an entirely insulated area from which drugs will be absent. Drugs are part of the world into which our children are growing up. They did not put them there. They are the result of a technological revolution, and the abuse of them is deeply rooted in adult society. It is simply absurd to imagine that we can keep young people away from them altogether. What we can do is to make sure that they are well-informed, that they are aware of the dangers and risks, and that they are sufficiently well integrated and 'together' that they will not seek through drugs a substitute for living.

This does not mean that vigilance is unnecessary, but it must be linked with trust and with common sense. Too much vigilance can lead to a suspicious spirit, a prying into our children's lives which betrays our lack of trust in them. Cases have been known where parents have sent their children's clothes to laboratories for analysis to detect traces of drugs on them. Once that stage has been reached, all human communication has broken down, and it is hardly surprising that the child seeks refuge in drugs. He is seeking refuge from his parents, and understandably so. It is essential that parents do not become detectives. However, provided that this is recognized, a reasonable degree of vigilance is right, and certain guidelines are useful.

The following are signs which are often associated with the use of certain drugs. *They need to be read with common sense, for many of the indications of drug misuse or abuse are hard to distinguish from ordinary adolescent mood changes. People often tell you to look for odd behaviour. But all adolescent behaviour is odd! Most of the signs of drug use can be reproduced by young people who have not been anywhere near drugs. So use the following list with caution.*

Cannabis

Cannabis is different from the other drugs in that it has a quite distinctive smell, rather like burning sage. Signs of its use are not very different from those of any other form of intoxication:

slow slurred speech;
excitability and inane laughter;
fatuous, dreamy expression;
flushed face;
relaxed but unsteady walk;
lack of interest in whatever is going on around;
wide glazed eyes.
Brown stains on the fingers, increased hunger and thirst with a preference for sweet food and drinks, dry cough, and reddening of the eyes may be observed.

Once it is known that an individual is using cannabis regularly, signs of deterioration *may* include the following;

difficulties in concentration;
failing memory;
decrease in mathematical ability;
a kind of 'creeping paranoia' with ideas of persecution;
exaggerated feelings either of self-confidence or inferiority;
passivity, loss of energy and desire;
difficulty in articulating thoughts and in expression;
increasing 'hang-ups' in close relationships especially with parents and with girl friends or boy friends;
increased impulsiveness and tendency to 'fly off the handle';
and a sense of futility and hopelessness about the future.

Amphetamines

The effects of amphetamine use have been referred to earlier. Signs of use may include:

restlessness and irritable behaviour;
alternating moods of elation and depression;
a 'bright-eyed' look combined with a lack of tact;
photophobia (fear of bright lights which hurt the eyes) and large pupils which may lead to the wearing of dark glasses; loss of appetite and weight, but increased thirst, dry mouth, and bad breath;
a tendency to sleep late on Mondays and to stay out all night.

Glue

See above (pp. 38–41) for details. It is worth noting here also that glue smells and causes sores round mouth and nose.

Opiates

The evidence of opiate use is more obvious. Changes in behaviour may be associated with a recent 'fix', or with the 'come down', or with the general way of life. Such signs as the following may be observed.

1   Changes associated with a recent 'fix'

Small pin-point pupils;
a dreamy and detached look;
fresh injection marks;
loss of appetite and of interest in food;
rubbing of eyes, chin and nose, and scratching of arms and legs;
slow and slurred speech;
resentfulness of being disturbed, and of noise and bright lights;

wakefulness interrupted by drowsiness;
eyes wide open but glazed, red and puffy;
relaxed posture;
constant examining of arms;
frequent visits to the lavatory;
inability to concentrate.

2   *Changes associated with a 'come down'*

Irritability, wanting to be left alone;
fidgeting with hands, pacing up and down;
inability to concentrate;
perspiration;
loss of appetite;
yawning;
running eyes and nose;
heavy smoking.

3   *Changes associated with way of life*

Blood spots on clothes, especially on pyjama tops and shirts;
unexpected absence from home;
sleeping out;
increased number of telephone calls and new visitors at home;
abandoning of organized activities;
poor appetite;
slow, halting speech;
loss of interest in personal appearance;
stooped posture;
long periods spent alone;
fully burnt matches found lying around;
litter in rooms and pockets.

It must be stressed again that it is the combination of these signs which, in a particular context, might lead one to believe that there is a drug-abuse problem. Taken in isolation, the signs may be due to a variety of factors, and one can get into positions and reach conclusions which are utterly ridiculous.

In general, it is more important to look for changes in behaviour than to look for drugs. But always remember that *virtually all drug effects can be produced without the use of drugs.* If you are genuinely worried and suspect that drugs may have caused the changes that you observe, it is best not to waste time thinking about it, but to take the simple method of *asking.*

Seeking help for yourself has already been stressed. There is always a danger that one sees the problem as residing in the other person. But we, as parents, are to a certain extent responsible for the situation which has arisen. We cannot pretend to be totally neutral, and we are, for better or worse, very involved. It is vital that we ensure that we receive adequate care and support, for without it we are likely to 'go under'. Yet so often we find that parents are worn to a frazzle by the pressure of events, and are in a very weak position to be of real help. To be concerned about one's own inner resources and one's sanity is not self-indulgence: it is common sense, and the exercise of proper responsibility. To inflict a weary, disintegrated person upon someone in deep distress is not compassionate but cruel and irresponsible.

Again, to emphasize a point made earlier, it is best to trust young people with information — and with life. It is not wise to treat them as small children, always to be preserved from the storms and tempests. Young people are much better at coping and surviving than we sometimes think. To protect them from harm can be twisted into protecting them from reality. The drug advice agency Release commented in 1976:

> With about nine years reactive experience of street drug crises we have encountered many problems which would not have occurred had people possessed some basic knowledge of the drug they were using. We feel it is important to provide information to children on request.

But it is not simply a matter of information. Young people need to feel able to talk to us about their feelings, their attitudes to drugs, and to life as a whole. If they are confronted by adult defensiveness and discomfort, they will see through it. So it is essential to listen, not to interrupt, to avoid sarcasm, preaching, and deliberate humiliation. The creation of a relaxed atmosphere in which problems can be worked through is the most valuable gift that parents can offer.

However, it needs to be stressed that no parent can do everything. We must accept out limitations. Young people are moving into the independence of adult life. To respect their individuality, to let them go, to trust them with life, is one of the most difficult lessons of being an adult. Children need to be protected from adult possessiveness and zeal for their welfare, for the wrong kind of 'help' can be more damaging than drugs. Kahlil Gibran, in *The Prophet*, expressed this in moving and profound words:

> You may give them your love but not your thoughts
> For they have their own thoughts.
> You may house their bodies but not their souls
> For their souls dwell in the house of tomorrow,
> Which you cannot visit, not even in your dreams.
> You may strive to be like them, but seek not to make them like you.
> For life goes not backward, nor tarries with yesterday.
> You are the bows from which your children as living arrows are sent forth.

Appendix 1

Resources for Further Help and Bibliography

A *Organizations and resources for information*

The most important source for all information relating to drug problems, facilities for help, and every aspect of the drug scene is the Institute for the Study of Drug Dependence, 3 Blackburn Road, London NW6 (01-328 5541). The Institute library covers the whole range of the field, and as well as books it contains a very large collection of journals, articles and press reports. The staff are extremely helpful and efficient, and are able to look up facts very quickly. People who wish to deepen their study of drug abuse are strongly advised to use the ISDD facilities and to subscribe to its valuable journal *Druglink* which keeps you up to date with developments.

At the same address is the Standing Conference on Drug Abuse (SCODA, 01-328 6556) which is also a very valuable source of information. SCODA publishes two important books: *Directory of Projects* and *Residential Rehabilitation Projects for Drug Dependents Referral Guide*. The Directory, published in collaboration with a number of other agencies, is a detailed guide to agencies and groups working in the drug field and related fields such as alcoholism, care of ex-offenders, and so on. The Referral Guide is an invaluable supplement to this, dealing specifically with facilities for treatment and after-care of addicts.

The following addresses are also useful:

Health Education Council, 78 New Oxford Street, London WC1A 1AH (01-637 1881)
Schools Council, 160 Great Portland Street, London W1N 6CC (01-580 0352)
TACADE (Teachers' Advisory Council on Alcohol and Drug

Education), 2 Mount Street, Manchester M25NG (061-834 7210)

Release (see below also), 1 Elgin Avenue, London W9 3PR (01-289 1123; 24-hour emergency service: 01-603 8654).

As a general rule, ISDD is the best source for literature, SCODA for guidance on facilities for help, and Release for the 'street-level' drug scene.

B *Bibliography*

The literature on drug use and abuse is enormous, and there are many thousands of books, pamphlets and articles. Below are listed books which are easy to obtain in Britain, which are not too technical for the general reader, and which deal in detail with aspects which have only been referred to briefly in this book. But they are a very small selection from a massive and growing area of study.

Sidney Cohen, *The Substance Abuse Problem* (New York, Haworth Press 1981) is one of the most comprehensive guides to drugs of abuse. Although it is written within the US context, much of it is equally applicable to Britain, and it should not be too difficult to obtain it here.

Griffith Edwards and Carol Busch have edited an excellent volume, *Drug Problems in Britain: A Review of Ten Years* (Academic Press 1981). This is a comprehensive survey and introduces the reader to much of the literature.

Ruth C. Engs, *Responsible Drug and Alcohol Use* (Collier-Macmillan 1979) is full of good, practical advice.

Jerome Jaffe, Robert Petersen and Ray Hodgson, *Addictions, Issues and Answers* (Harper and Row 1980) is well-produced and very well illustrated.

Peter Laurie, *Drugs: Medical, Psychological and Social Facts* (Penguin, 1978 edn) has now gone through several editions and revisions, and is one of the best introductions to the field.

Richard R. Lingeman, *Drugs from A to Z: A Dictionary* (McGraw-Hill 1969) is excellent.

Peter Parish, *Medicines: A Guide for Everybody* (Penguin, 1980 edn), written by one of Britain's experts on drug prescribing, covers a much wider area than drug abuse. This book deals with the whole question of the use of drugs in medicine.

M.A. Plant, *Drugs in Perspective* (Teach Yourself Books 1981) is a sober, cautious and unemotional survey of our present state of knowledge. Plant is one of the most careful students of the subject.

Anthony Ryle, *Student Casualties* (Penguin 1969) has a section on drugs, but the whole book is relevant to the pressures on young people at college.

There is a considerable literature on specific drugs. Perhaps the best introduction to the present state of knowledge on cannabis is J.D.P. Graham, *Cannabis Now* (H.M.& M.Publishers Ltd, Milton Road, Aylesbury, Bucks, 1977). Graham is a leading pharmacologist and one of the international authorities on cannabis. On LSD and the psychedelics, Lester Grinspoon and James B. Bakalar, *Psychedelic Drugs Reconsidered* (New York, Basic Books 1979) is an up-to-date and useful study. On glue, see Eve Merrill, *Glue Sniffing: a guide for professionals, and parents* (from ISDD).

There are few books addressed directly to children, and those which do exist are often patronizing and inaccurate. Perhaps the best of those available at present is Fiona Foster and Alexander McCall Smith, *So You Want to Try Drugs?* (Loanhead, Midlothian 1980). For teenagers — and others — the various pamphlets published by Release are probably the best and most respected sources of information. They include:

Drugs: a brief factual guide
Sniffing glue and other solvents

Legal drugs (alcohol and tobacco)
Cannabis
Amphetamines
Heroin and other opiates

Most books on poisoning emergencies and overdose are designed for medical staff, but some can be usefully read by the lay person. Two books which are of help are Peter A. Czajka and James P.Duffy, *Poisoning Emergencies* (The C.V.Mosby Company, St Louis, Toronto and London, 1980) and Gordon Matthews and Sue James, *Coping with Drugs*: *Rational Responses to their Use* (Cyrenians, 13 Wincheap, Canterbury, CT1 3TB, 1975).

A good legal approach is David Farrier, *Drugs and Intoxication* (Sweet and Maxwell, Modern Legal Studies, 1980).

Appendix 2

Drugs and the Law

Most of the drugs which are used are subject to minimal controls (e.g. alcohol, barbiturates) or no controls at all (e.g. glue). But drugs such as cannabis, LSD, heroin and others are controlled by the Misuse of Drugs Act 1971. The possession of barbiturates is not an offence, but sale without a prescription is prohibited under the Medicines Act 1968.

The Misuse of Drugs Act divides controlled drugs into three categories:

Class A includes cocaine, heroin, LSD, morphine, methadone, PCP, and a number of opiates, synthetic narcotic and hallucinogens, and also amphetamines when prepared for injection.

Class B includes amphetamine, cannabis, codeine, DF 118, Preludin and Ritalin.

Class C includes methaqualone (Mandrax) and some stimulants.

The following are the maximum penalties in a Crown Court under the Act:

	Possession	*Possession with intent to supply; and Supply*
Class A	7 years or unlimited fine	14 years or unlimited fine.
Class B	5 years or unlimited fine	5 years or unlimited fine
Class C	2 years or unlimited fine	5 years or unlimited fine.

For more details see the leaflet *Drugs and the Law* obtainable from Release, 1 Elgin Avenue, London W9 3PR.

A Short Glossary of Drug Slang

Many of these words are now integrated into mainstream English. However, some of them are still unfamiliar, and it is felt that they should be included. But it is important not to be misled by a glossary into thinking that drug abuse is an esoteric, private world where even the language is alien. It should also be noted that terms vary from time to time and from place to place. The following list contains only the commonly used terms.

Acid	LSD
Amp	ampoule, a drug container, usually containing methadone
Black bombers	20 milligramme capsule of Durophet (amphetamine)
Blues	Drinamyl tablet (amphetamine barbiturate compound)
Bread	money
Buzz	immediate pleasant effect of drug
Bum trip	bad experience of LSD; also applied to events
Coke	cocaine
Cold turkey	coming off heroin without the aid of substitute drugs.
Come down	to lose the drug effect as it wears off
Crash out; Crash	to pass out, go to sleep, after drug use
Crash pad	temporary place to sleep
Deal	drug transaction

Fix	to inject a drug
Freak out	a psychedelic happening or event; also to go 'out of your mind' through a drug experience; used loosely to mean a wild time
Fuzz	police
Grass	marijuana
H	heroin
Habit	amount of a drug needed for satisfaction
Head	originally anyone using drugs (acidhead, pillhead, etc.), but also loosely applied (e.g. bread-head = money grubber)
High	feeling good, euphoria
Hooked	addicted
Jack up	inject heroin or other drug
Joint	cannabis cigarette
Junk	heroin or related drug
Junkie	person addicted to heroin or other injectible drug
Kick	to stop taking drugs
Mainline	to inject drugs
Pillhead	an amphetamine user
Score	to obtain drugs
Script	prescription
Shit	cannabis resin
Shoot	inject
Smack	heroin

A SHORT GLOSSARY OF DRUG SLANG

Speed	amphetamine
Stoned	in a happy drugged condition
Trip	experience with LSD; also used loosely to describe any experience
Turn on	to smoke cannabis; to introduce a person to drugs
Weed	marijuana

Index

Overcoming Common Problems
MAIL ORDER FORM

ARTHRITIS *Dr William Fox*   £1.50 ☐
  Is your suffering really necessary

BIRTH OVER THIRTY *Sheila Kitzinger*   £2.50 ☐

ENJOYING MOTHERHOOD *Dr Brice Pitt*   £1.95 ☐
  How to have a happy pregnancy

THE EPILEPSY HANDBOOK *Shelagh McGovern*   £3.95 ☐

FEARS AND PHOBIAS *Dr Tony Whitehead*   £1.95 ☐

FEELING HEALTHY *Dr F. E. Kenyon*   £1.95 ☐
  How to stop worrying about your health

GUILT *Dr Vernon Coleman*   £1.95 ☐

HERPES *Dr Oscar Gillespie*   £3.95 ☐

HOW TO CONTROL YOUR DRINKING *Dr Miller & Dr Munoz*
                                                              £3.95 ☐

HOW TO COPE WITH STRESS *Dr Peter Tyrer*   £1.95 ☐

HOW TO COPE WITH YOUR NERVES *Dr Tony Lake*   £2.50 ☐

HOW TO SLEEP BETTER *Dr Peter Tyrer*   £1.95 ☐

LONELINESS *Dr Tony Lake*   £1.95 ☐

MEETING PEOPLE IS FUN *Dr Phyllis Shaw*   £1.95 ☐
  How to overcome shyness

MAKING THE MOST OF MIDDLE AGE *Dr Brice Pitt*   £1.95 ☐

NO MORE HEADACHES *Lilian Rowen*   99p ☐

OVERCOMING TENSION *Dr Kenneth Hambly*   £1.95 ☐

ONE PARENT FAMILIES *Diana Davenport*   £2.95 ☐
  A practical guide to coping

SELF-HELP FOR YOUR ARTHRITIS *Edna Pemble*   £1.95 ☐

THE SEX ATLAS *Dr Erwin Haeberle*   £10   ☐

STRESS AND YOUR STOMACH *Dr Vernon Coleman*   £1.95 ☐

SUCCESSFUL SEX *Dr F. E. Kenyon*   £1.95 ☐

WHAT EVERYONE SHOULD KNOW ABOUT DRUGS
Kenneth Leech   £2.50 ☐

By Dr Paul Hauck

CALM DOWN   £2.50 ☐
  How to cope with frustration and anger

DEPRESSION   £1.95 ☐

HOW TO BRING UP YOUR CHILD SUCCESSFULLY   £2.95 ☐

HOW TO DO WHAT YOU WANT TO DO   £1.95 ☐

HOW TO STAND UP FOR YOURSELF   £1.95 ☐

JEALOUSY   £2.50 ☐

MAKING MARRIAGE WORK   £1.95 ☐

WHY BE AFRAID?   £1.95 ☐
  How to overcome your fears

All these books can be ordered direct by post. Just tick the titles you want and fill in the form below.

Name ....

Address ....

....

....

Write to OCP Mail Order, SPCK, Marylebone Road, London NW1 4DU. Please enclose remittance to the value of the cover price plus:
UK: 50p for the first book plus 30p per copy for each additional book ordered.
Overseas: 75p for the first book plus 45p per copy for each additional book.

Sheldon Press reserve the right to show new retail prices on covers which may differ from those previously advertised in the text or elsewhere. Postage rates are also subject to revision.